Printed in the United States of America

First Printing, 2020

ISBN 978-0-578-69397-2

Sparkle Communications LLC
Palm Beach, Fl 33480

www.marygiuseffi.com

# Acknowledgements

Undeniably You is proof positive that when extraordinary, talented, gorgeous souls unite in a vision to uplift each other and support one voice, miracles happen. Thank you to each of the spirit filled amazing people who believed in this project and generously shared their talent with me and you in the creation of this book.

To the thousands of women who I have been honored and privileged to dress and who have allowed me to see their vulnerability and beauty-thank you. You are truly packaged to perfection... so grateful for the experiences of creating your visual brands and wardrobes for your best lives.

To my exquisite ubiquitous and undeniable beauty girl, my daughter Gina... your love, candor, clarity, commitment, talent and tenacity made my dreams come true. Thank you for every moment- your love is like no other.... how blessed am I to have you in my life and heart. Your creative genius solved the seemingly unsolvable problems in manifesting Undeniably You! Thank you.

To my incredibly talented, generous and ingenious, funny and fantastic, creative artists - my illustrators, Robin and Tracey, friends for life. Thank you for painting the most fabulous renderings and reading my mind and heart. You rushed in where angels feared to tread. Without your faith and hard work, Undeniably You would have remained just a dream.

Thank you to Mimi, for pouring your enormous talent, creativity and gracious spirit into this book. Your art direction and design so perfectly manifested my vision.... you are a joy and your friendship makes my heart and the world smile!

To my Champagne Sisters, Andrea, Diana and Debbie, who lift me up, roll up their sleeves, lean it, and believe, against all odds, that this voice needs to be heard. You are the wind beneath my wings and the bubbles in my bubbly! Pop, Fizz, Clink! I love you! Thank you!

To Ish Major ... there are no words to describe what it is like to walk side by side on this extraordinary journey of becoming who we are.... thank you for your love and joy...for your guidance and glistening soul... thank you for lifting women up on their journeys to live their highest and best lives every day and showing up as an advocate love and healing. Thank you for penning the most exquisite forward to this book. I am eternally grateful for you!

Thank you to my colleague and dear friend, Steve, marketing and publicity master, for pouring decades of wisdom, expertise and guidance into my being. You, Laura, Geoffrey and your team have made and make all the difference on so many levels. Deep gratitude to you for shining your light on this project! And special thanks to Cristina for your wisdom and insights.

To my mentors and the visionaries for my life, my Grandmother and Mother... you are with me every day... thank you for fiercely protecting your little girl and for teaching me everything there is to know about life, love and fashion.

To my granddaughter Arielle... the world is your stage, your brilliance and enthusiasm, talent and tenacity will make the entire globe sing! NaNa loves you with all her heart! You and your friends are the future fashionistas. I rest gratefully and confidently in your precious hands!

And for all my family and grandchildren, thank you for always standing by me and supporting my mission. David... there is no one like you my precious son and confidante... your compassion and courage soothe and save hurting people... and your heart, faith, loyalty and love make every day the best day of my life.

Andreas, thank you for your love and generosity, guidance, and constancy. All of our dreams come true because of you. You so encourage this Champagne Girl to trust her wings and fly! I love you!

And to my Divine Creator.... love is all.... thank you for every day and for guiding my every step. God is good all the time.

*Mary Ginseffi*

# Forward: By Dr. Ish Major

What you have in your hands at this very moment contains some of the most personally empowering tools that are available to you. And I should know, because I've had the privilege of using them personally. The tools she's about to give you are the very tools she gave me and they, along with Mary's indomitable spirit is the very reason I'm able to write this foreword fully ensconced from my Reality TV catbird seat standing firm in the knowledge that wherever this ride takes me I'll show up fully garbed, fully armed and wholly me.

Some things in life are a no-brainer; Mary Giuseffi is one of them. One of the things that make this book so unique is that Mary is one of the few true experts who's speaking and teaching from an authentic perspective. She can teach it because she's lived it. We have so many 'experts' these days that can give you the full benefit of everything they've read and surmised...but precious few who can give you the full benefit of what they've manifested. If your guru du jour hasn't done the things you are trying to do then you need a new guru.

My life changed the day I met Mary. She taught me how to say "Yes!" to myself and "Yes!" to the life that was waiting for me! And from that fateful day until this one, I've never looked back! I'm writing this foreword because of my unique perspective about Mary. I've had the distinct advantage of having her work with me. I've had the privilege of her pouring her knowledge, wisdom and belief into me. I now experience the glory of living the manifestations of that belief every day. I'll never forget the first words Mary ever said to me. She took one look at me and said, "You've got it!" And I was off and running from there! The power of belief that comes from someone who has a knowing is truly astounding.

Freedom, ultimate freedom, is the privilege of showing up in the world exactly as who you are. Imagine if when you did, the world not only accepted you for it, it actually loved you because of it! That's the gift of freedom Mary is here to give to you! And if you're not quite ready to apply what's within these pages that's ok too. Simply keep the book close. Read a few excerpts here and there while you wrap your mind around the idea of re-wrapping your body anew. Mary is boundless joy and that energy permeates this book. Keep it close long enough and that same feeling will permeate that inner formless energy that is you and when you're ready, it will show you how to show up in your world fully formed!

Motivation is letting the things you want drive you forward. Inspiration is allowing who you are to call you forward. In that same vein, Mary is inspiring you to new heights. She's calling you forward. The only question is; are you ready to answer.

We all have that inner voice. That true self. It's that untouched and untapped energy that that makes you uniquely you that has remained pure from day one until day now. The problem is the world throws so many roadblocks and distractions our way it's easy to lose sight of it. If you go long enough without seeing it you may even start to believe it's no longer there. And nothing could be further from the truth! In the pages of this book you'll find a re-awakening of that place. You'll get back into conscious contact with that endless stream of boundless energy and limitless joy that is you! That place of well-being is where you came from. It's not a place you have to work to find your way back to. It's simply a place you have to remember, close your eyes and allow it to find you; again.

This book is so much more than about wardrobe and style and fashion. It's about fashioning your life into the masterpiece that it was meant to be.

I've sat at the feet of the masterful presence that is Mary Giuseffi. I've had the honor of knowing her personally for 10 years. We've had countless conversations about life an love and joy, so you can take it from when I tell you this much is true—you're about to go on a journey that will truly change your life—being guided by one of the most authentic women and genuine spirits I've ever seen. I would encourage you to not only read the words in this book but also take a moment to sit with what she's teaching you and then immediately apply it to your life. Your world will change right before your very eyes. And not only is that what you want, it's what your true self wants for you!

I called Mary the day I booked my first big TV gig and I'll never forget what she told me. She said, "Ish, dreams do to come true! And this is only the beginning!" And I've never known her to be wrong!

Thank you Mary for the honor of saying a few words in your amazing work.

Thank you, MORE!

*Dr. Ish Major*

Dr. Ish Major
The Host of WeTV's Hit Series Marriage Bootcamp Reality Stars
One Of America's Top Psychiatrists
Author and Dating Expert

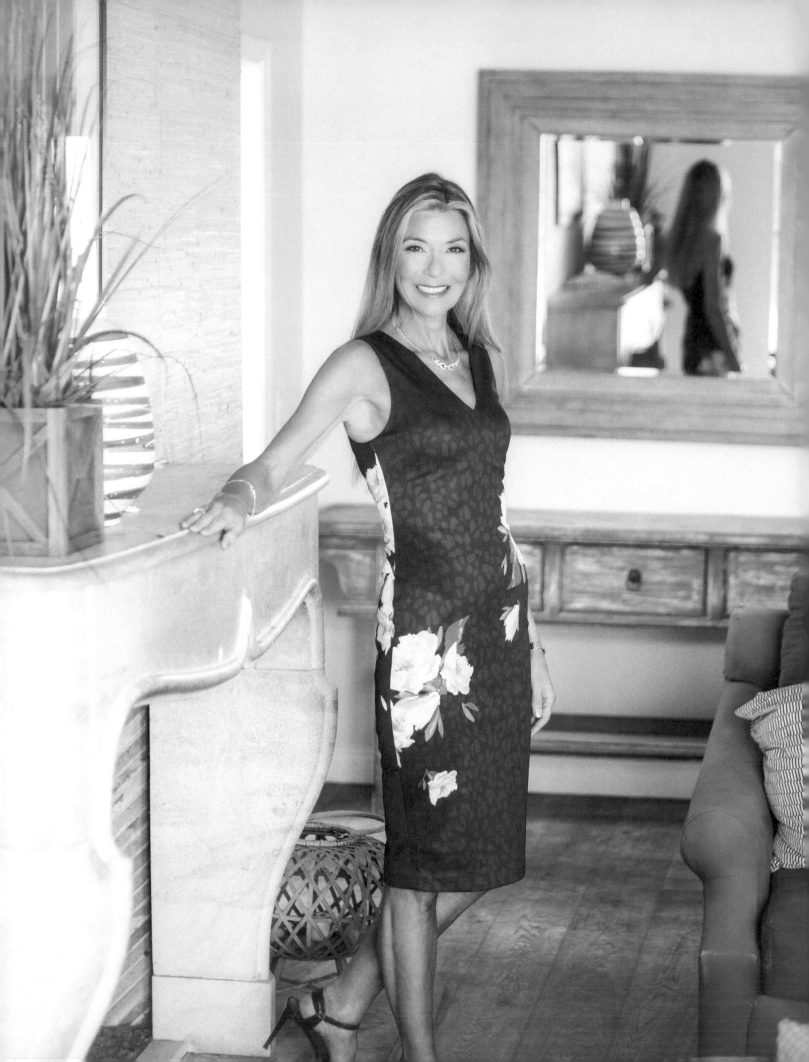

# *Introduction*

So, what can I say, I'm just a girl from New Jersey who wanted to change the world one outfit at a time. The crazy thing is that in spite of myself and my passion for fashion, opera, bad boys and Champagne, my crazy over the top life, with its spectacular triumphs and tragedies, has left me still standing in stilettos with my bubbles, baubles, beau du jour and beatific vision intact!

I mean, what's a nice girl to do? I went from riches to rags to riches so many times that there were days I couldn't remember who I was and got dressed in my bygone days closet riches to play out my current secret life as bag lady in rags. It was survival in two gears: couture princess in public and a "homeless" person in private. People thought that I was a trust fund baby waiting for my car or a waiflike pan handler at the airport. It was nobody's business. It was survival of the fittest… outfit. My self-esteem was bereft, food budget might have been three dollars a day but my image looked like a million. When you've tripped the light fantastic for a living… you either end up with bruises or badges and dearests I have my share of both!

What kept me afloat and sane, ok, that is questionable, when the going got tough was my gift for garb! My pedigreed knowledge for fashion and instinctual awareness of how to make a girl sparkle was my money shot! I really knew my way around a department store, an audition and a cocktail party. More than anything, I loved to see women feel like a million bucks in their clothes. Thousands of miles in malls and thousands of satisfied grown up and gorgeous clients later, I am proud to say it all worked out sublimely. I am the shopping Contessa for a cause…. delivering the goods from my home to yours!

I've realized that Some days are too good to be true, some days are so bad that you cannot even admit it to yourself. As long as you show up looking fabulous… an Undeniably You, you will triumph as a model citizen, in the end! God does bless the girl that has her own… wardrobe, style and savvy.

*Cheers to making dreams your come true. Let's get dressed!*

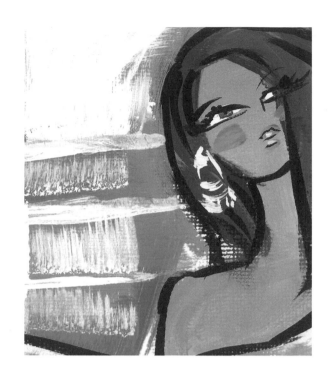

# Undeniably You!

## The Good, the Bad and the Fabulous!

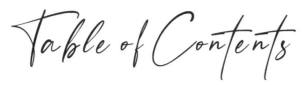
# Table of Contents

1.  Fashion Forward "The Dressing Room".............................................. 14

2.  How to Use This Book .............................................................. 20

3.  Your Guide to Authentic Style .................................................... 24

4.  Which Archetypal Personality Are You? ............................................ 30

5.  The Maverick ..................................................................... 32

6.   The Icon ........................................................................ 36

7.  The Angelic ...................................................................... 40

8.  The Creative ..................................................................... 44

9.  The Innocent ..................................................................... 48

10. The Alchemist .................................................................... 52

11. The Lover ........................................................................ 56

12. What Is Your Style Persona? ...................................................... 60

13. The Entrance Maker ............................................................... 64

14. The Eternal Beauty ............................................................... 70

15. The Explorer Naturalist .......................................................... 76

16. The Hopeful Romantic ............................................................. 82

17. The Carefree Casual .............................................................. 88

18. The Bohemian Rhapsody ............................................................ 94

19. The Energetic Sprite ............................................................ 100

20. The Ingenue Muse ................................................................ 106

21. The Combination Style Personas and Summary ..................................... 112

22. It's Sort of Like Champagne ..................................................... 116

23. A Frame by Any Other Name ....................................................... 124

24. Loving the Skin You're In ....................................................... 138

25. Your Divine Colors .............................................................. 156

26. The Gentle Art of Color Persuasion ............................................. 192

27. How Line, Color, and Shape Can Be Your Best Fashion Influencers ....200

28. Wardrobe Capsule Dressing ....................................................... 206

29. The Finale ...................................................................... 214

# CHAPTER 1

## Fashion Forward: The Dressing Room

As I sit here, writing about how seamless your second skin experience should be in life, I am writing this book in my first skin. Every summer, my beau and I return to paradise found, his little cottage on the Atlantic coast of France. It is unfettered and unembellished. Far from a runway of any kind, it is a naturist camp. So, as I share with you my passion for fashion and my lifelong pursuit of creating beauty in form, fit, fabric in love and joy, it's sort of funny that I am writing in the nude. Hopefully, my insights and thoughts will give you some sound advice for creating your best formula for dressing and feeling your best.

To that point, I will offer this premise: if you are not comfortable in your first skin, it is hard to find happiness in your second skin.

Clothing is not meant to camouflage your faults and hide your deep secrets; it exists to do the exact opposite. Fashion exists to celebrate your uniqueness and express your personal mission to the world. I am always amazed when I arrive here how comfortable people are in their bodies. The layers of self-consciousness and self-judgment seem to vanish as the cultural mores that hold us hostage in our wardrobe wear thin and, all at once, utterly disappear. Young children run free or hop on skateboards and bikes, old people walk happily with their beach towels and baskets of bread and wine and cheese...tall, short, thin, thick, wrinkled, brand new...each person seems so unafraid and unconcerned with anyone else's thoughts about their bodies or their beings. They are not even preoccupied by their profile or rear view. They are present and accounted for. They are alive and well. What a lovely way to live.

The relationship we have with our naked being should be one of love and acceptance, not hatred and self-loathing. It is our vehicle for life; it doesn't define us...it provides us access to our physical world. Our bodies catalyze our thoughts and feelings, embody our soul, and demonstrate our will in time. Our bodies make our dreams come true. They are our temple...our divine partnership with life. Unfortunately, most of us have a love/hate relationship with our bodies and then wonder why we never seem to find anything we like to wear. I can't tell you how many times I have heard "I have a closet full of clothes and nothing to wear. I never feel good in my clothes." So, let me ask you, do you feel any better without your clothes?

## Hmmm... that's what I thought

My goal for you is to be as happy without clothes as you will be in clothes. Once we create for you your formula for dressing as your authentic selves and learn how to leverage your wardrobe in such a perfect and powerful way, your life will be transformed. By saying "yes" to the dress...or the pants or the shoes...you will enhance and elevate your life. Fall in love. Get a promotion. Create the company. Be paid what you're worth. Saying "yes" to your dress means saying "yes" to your life and achieving the success as only you can. My goal is that by creating a fashionable and actionable wardrobe, you will feel extraordinary and be inspired to embrace your passions and manifest your dream come true! Sound impossible? I think not. If you really want to see transformation, step into my dressing room.

I have witnessed miracles. I have seen women cry, not because they hate how they look but because for the first time in their lives, they love how they look. Countless women show up in my dressing room as passive-aggressive, indifferent-caring refugees seeking asylum and soul-utions to their wardrobe debacles. They rawly share nightmarish self-image confessions and stories about their failed relationships. They share all their "wills and will nots, never and only," exposing all the things they hate about their figures and the reasons why they look the way they do.

Reinforced by Instagram and retouched selfies, emotions are triggered.

"Whenever I see that color I think of...."

"My last boyfriend said he cheated on me because of my weight."

"Kids always made fun of me when I wore...."

"They said I was so fat my thighs rubbed together."

"I know I'm smart but if I just wore this tighter and shorter, I think I could get that job."

No, you might get a date, dear sister, but the job is a different story. Let's have enough confidence in our ability to secure your position. I say, "Okay, I understand and accept

*My goal is that by creating a fashionable and actionable wardrobe, you will feel extraordinary and be inspired to embrace your passions and manifest your dream come true!*

how you feel. So many women have felt this way. I have found that it is totally normal to feel that way.... Let's just try on this outfit! You don't have to buy it. You don't have to like it. Just do it for me so that I can see for myself where to go from here with your wardrobe."

Little by little, in front of me and behind closed doors, the truth shows its face. Then we can begin to disassemble the mythology of who a woman thinks she is, was told she is, and needs to be and assemble and honor who and what she truly is...a gorgeous soul having a totally human experience translated by a piece of cloth.

Slowly but surely, with every new piece a woman tries on, a piece of her authentic soul shows up. Slowly she rids herself of the misbeliefs and biases that were passed down to her by her mother and best friends. Little by little, the insecurities vanish as her story unfolds, her heart opens, and her light shines. Item by item... we can heal the painful experiences of her past. We can fix the fashion faux pas and wardrobe malfunctions and recreate a healthier, more loving experience for her future.

I have worked with transformationalists all my life. I went to the New School in the '70s as a psychology major and studied spiritual psychology in a well-known master's program. I have been Rolfed, reborn, rebalanced, renewed and restored, elevated and elongated, and connected, kundalinied, and Houdinied...and after all these years, I have come to this conclusion:

You want to see real transformation? I'll show you real transformation. It doesn't happen in an ashram or a chapel; it happens in a dressing room. Real transformation will begin the minute you step out of your imposter shell, get naked to the truth about your body and your life, and start wearing and being your authentic self. Exposed and "ex parte'ed." Transformation will occur when your second skin is true to your soul. Transformation occurs when we start saying "I love you" instead of "I hate you" while

> *"I have witnessed miracles.*
> *I have seen women cry, not because*
> *they hate how they look*
> *but because for the first time*
> *in their lives,*
> *they love how they look."*

gazing in the mirror. That, my beautiful friends, is transformation. The rest will follow. Let's begin by wearing the dress that makes you feel like the queen and the diviner of your destiny. Let's start by saying "yes" to life and to a new wardrobe that communicates exactly who you are to the world in the highest and best manner.

Women love makeovers, queen for a day, bachelorette, talent shows as well as beauty contests. We love the underdog and can't resist a little campiness and bravado. Welcome to your makeover. Let's agree on this: This is your moment. This is your show. The Big Reveal is you.

# CHAPTER 2
## *How to Use This Book*

There are thousands of fashion and style blogs, articles, and books on the market today. My wish is for you to never need to read another book, take another quiz, or view another video on trying to figure out who you are in fashion. My hope for you is that this book will provide you with enough information, understanding, and courage to discover and embody your core persona and be successful in defining that style for the world. It is a comprehensive introduction to creating Undeniably YOU!

There are many sections and many subjects to cover. This is not exhaustive but rather an exhilarating cumulative approach to self-discovery. Each chapter will highlight a topic and present an overview for your edification. Each chapter will offer advice and assistance in understanding the tricks of the trade and the secrets of a lifetime fashionista cum clairvoyant cum stylist. I have created a formula to guide you on your way out of the dressing room and onto your personal runway.

Each of us longs for a feeling of community belongingness, being understood and able to express ourselves authentically in the world, seamlessly conveying our passions and purpose every day to specific audiences from our loved ones to our clients and society at large. Our second skin should not only be like us; it should behave, feel and speak for us the minute we enter a room.

The objective of this book is to assist you in understanding who you are authentically and how to create a wardrobe that celebrates and supports you at every moment, in a million different environments. It should amplify the aspects of your being that should be called forward, while protecting those aspects that are reserved for private, intimate moments. The perfect wardrobe should serve as your opening conversation, your business card, your armor, your companion, your confidante. It should define who you are, why you are here, what you want to accomplish, and what you bring to the table, and express your assets and priorities. Your wardrobe predicts your relationship with others. If it describes you well, your relationships will develop successfully and bring you happiness forever after... So, what do you think? Let's party!

In order to truly step into an empowered, limitless potential, you first have to create your ideal stage, emotionally connecting with your envisioned future, experiencing it before it happens. Clothes are an extraordinary and wholly visceral vehicle for connecting someone to her source, providing absolute clarity and affirmation regarding a limitless potential for the future! Visualization and meditation set the stage for manifesting your potential.

If you believe that you can truly attain your career and life goals and are committed to the process of becoming, you must first create a personal style that vibrates at that level every day, signaling not only to the world but to yourself that this potentiality already exists for you in the world. All that you want to be must be seen in your vision board. Your wardrobe should reflect your personality, embody your passion to show up as your authentic self—even if you are in transition, or at the very beginning of your growth and development. The mirror should reflect, proof positive, an image of the finished product of who you are in the process of becoming. Seeing is believing. If you see yourself sexy, successful, and satisfied, you will feel fabulous. You will create positive and loving emotional self-beliefs and in doing so shift your entire energetic soul print to being the finished product! Changing your outfit will transform your life!

*"Once you follow my formula for creating an image and a lifestyle that is Undeniably You, be prepared for manifesting the life that you deserve."*

*"Pop! Fizz! Clink! You are about to step into your big girl shoes and make the world your runway."*

Here is how we are going to discover your authentic self, inside and out:

1.  Discover your archetypal personality and authentic nature.
2.  Define your style personality.
3.  Determine your body type and frame your physical being.
4.  Delve into your divine colors and describe your soul's mission.
5.  Display a visual seasonal energy field that is in alignment with your coloring and optimizes your potential.
6.  Delineate, raise and refine your vibration to match your ideal self.
7.  Design a wardrobe that embodies and portrays to the world who you are, what you want, and how you will impact the planet by raising the world's vibration with your unique gifts, talents, passions, and abilities.

Once you have a firm grasp on all this powerful information, party on and:

8.  Explore your image as art.
9.  Experience how to shop like a stylist.
10. Explode onto the runway in your style DNA platform.
11. Become Undeniably You!

And then, we shall pop, fizz, clink, and celebrate your success and enjoy the after-party!

Once you follow my formula for creating an image and a lifestyle that is Undeniably You, be prepared for manifesting the life that you deserve. Yes! You are about to step into your big girl shoes and make the world your runway. Don't worry if you don't finish the book. It is intended to be an evergreen guide to grow your fabulousness and embrace your ever-changing, transformational life journey. Do not get too bogged down with the details or frustrated by the process. The key is this: Believe in the miracle that is you at the core. Embrace your undeniable self. Stake your claim. Invest in your best and discard all the rest! Are you ready for the world to witness your entrance on to any stage you aspire to own and claim as your own? Let's do this, girls…. I am here for you every step of the way!

# CHAPTER 3

*Your Guide to Authentic Style*

When I think about how women dress, there are certain women that stand out: the risk takers, the play-it-safers, the sheer rebels, the hot messes, the iconoclasts, the recyclers...most of us fall somewhere in between. Twice a year, spring and fall, we feverishly attempt to become "on trend," adapting our style to something we see in a magazine or on social media. A trip to the mall later, discouraged and depressed, we wind up wearing a new version of the same old stuff, hiding behind our clothes instead of allowing the clothes to showcase who we are authentically, in our world today. Dressing becomes a herculean and self-sabotaging task. Our self-esteem is found on the closet floor where we left all our discarded hopes and dreams. Frustrated and confused, we opt to wear our "uniform." It's not great. It's not really me. But it will have to do.

## Creating Your Personal Brand

A few years ago, I was invited to do a segment on branding for the Today Show. I came up with this simple formula:

## *How You Look + How You Act + How You Speak = Your Personal Brand.*

Your personal brand is reflected in the way your image is received. It is your commercial to the world. We all have one running. What does your commercial say about you?

What are your beliefs? What are your passions? What are your responsibilities? How do you spend your days? Who do you encounter along the way? What do you want to share? What do you want to reveal about yourself? What are your goals? Your personal brand and visual grammar should convey this with confidence, clarity, and direction. Your wardrobe should send a focused message to the viewer of how you want to be treated. It should reveal your best attributes. Your appearance should give you a five-star rating. It should positively impact your chosen environment and public opinion.

## Visual Language and First Impressions

Creating an intentional, authentic visual language frees us from immediate and long-lasting judgment. It announces us before we speak and conveys our brand and mission to the world. Studies have shown that it takes less than 1/10th of a second to form a first impression. It is almost entirely visual. Once that perception is formed, it may take an eternity to change. Opinions, good, bad, or fabulous, stick like glue. It's time to harness that power and create an image that truly introduces you to the world with an empowered real statement.

Our culture, our demographic, and our paycheck also factor into our visual language. Our style consciousness reveals our rootedness in the past and willingness to embrace future potential. Have you ever seen a woman who is trapped in "her most beautiful period"? She is still wearing the same makeup and hair from her most beloved decade. Sadly, time has marched on and she has been left with a face she cannot recognize without her armor. Although she appears totally dated, she refuses to update her look because she is convinced that she is still that young beautiful thing. We are not forever young. The eyeliner doesn't help. Opting for a new look will create a youthful and more attractive appearance. She is stuck. Aren't we all from time to time?

## The 4 R's

When we talk about selecting wardrobe for a visual brand or a style consciousness, there are four factors to consider:

Am I relatable?
Am I relevant?
Am I reliant?
Do I establish immediate rapport?

Nonverbal communication is a powerful way to create and solidify a relationship with a client, colleague, customer, friend, or significant other. Since a first impression is formed in less than 1/10th of a second, and the average time a person spends determining your value to them is less than seven seconds in the virtual world, your wardrobe choice is among the most important factors in creating a viable business

> *"It's time to harness that power and create an image that truly introduces you to the world with an empowered real statement."*

opportunity, being hired, making a sale, and getting a promotion. It is also an impactful way to attract and sustain personal relationships. Recent studies sadly show that appearance-based discrimination is alive and well, claiming that appearance influences client perception and company image up to 90%, employee confidence up to 85%, and competency as high as 73%. We may have come a long way, baby, but the world is still lagging behind.

People are more likely to trust and do business with someone who resembles themselves. They want to work with people who appear to share a similar worldview, background, belief system, lifestyle, and taste. People trust the familiar. Clothing can increase your likability. People hire people whom they like. They buy things from people who share a similar opinion. They trust someone who reflects their own values. They like to associate with people who make them feel comfortable and have a commonality of experience and feelings.

Your outfit conveys all this to the viewer. It not only creates a positive atmosphere, it offers an invitation to connect on an emotional level and establishes immediate rapport. "She likes what I like... yes, I like that woman. Let's work together! Let's buy a house from her." If you're outfit intimidates your potential client or is too overpowering in any way, a person's immediate reaction will be negative. "Oh! She doesn't understand me. We have nothing in common—she can't help me solve my problem. She has no idea how I feel." Relatability is key. It's all in the clothes!

Your clothing will also communicate your relevance in a group or one on one. Dressing in an updated and current way emits the message of relevance. The right piece says, "I'm on top of my game. I know exactly what's happening now, and I am here to bring you the latest technology, service, and product to assist you in living your best life."

In personal relationships, clothing can pre-determine your tribe and your romances. Out-of-date clothing makes you appear and feel out of date. No one wants last year's solutions to this year's problem. Update your look. Stay informed. Be current. Be articulate. The right garment reveals your self-mastery. Your modern approach to dressing informs your client that you have a modern mind. Your outfit influences their opinion regarding your competency and ability. It paves the way for an intellectual connection.

Establishing trust is imperative in any relationship, personal or professional. Reliance and trust can be easily established when your outfit expresses professionalism, timeliness, attention to detail, and strong moral values. Are you trustworthy? If you look trustworthy people are more likely to hire you. Trust is instinctual. And can be communicated as simply as selecting the appropriate-colored dress, lipstick, and shoes.

## How I A-Dress Myself

**The Before and After Quiz**

Guilty! When I see a personality test online or in a magazine, I am compelled to take it—aren't you? Who knows, it may provide a few insights. Since I am here to please, and totally raise my hand to the "tell me more about me" fascination, here is a quiz for you. I want you to take it twice—once before you read the book and once after you finish the book—and create your formula for becoming Undeniably You!

Please don't spend too time on this Q&A. There are no right or wrong answers. It is merely an assessment to mark the beginning and ending of your journey here, recognizing all the progress you will make along the way. Be honest with yourself. I am asking for your thoughts and feelings because it will provide a contrast and comparison and coax your inner fabulous self to remember the beautiful soul who is tucked inside and waiting to be seen and celebrated.

*"Reliance and trust can be easily established when your outfit expresses professionalism, timeliness, attention to detail, and strong moral values."*

# Q&A

*When I look in the mirror today, this is how I A-Dress myself...*

I am _____

I keep _____

I wish I could _____

I love _____

I dance when _____

I sing to _____

I think _____

I really wish that _____

I need _____

I should _____

I can _____

I like _____

I make _____

I always _____

If I could change one thing _____

The one thing, I wish people knew about me _____

I am here to _____

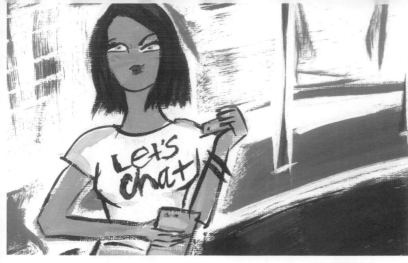

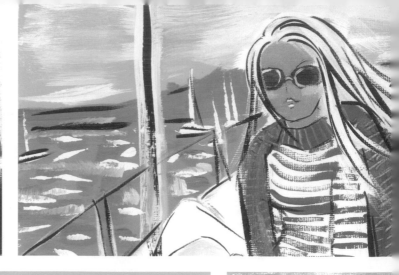

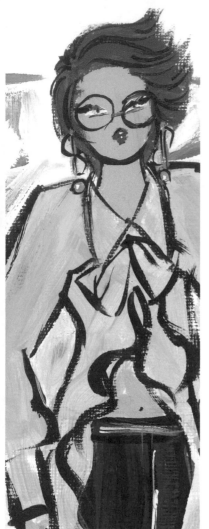

Each woman is
described by her
Defining Qualities, Life
Mission and Vision,
and Authentic Style
Language.

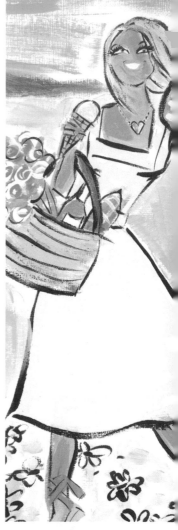

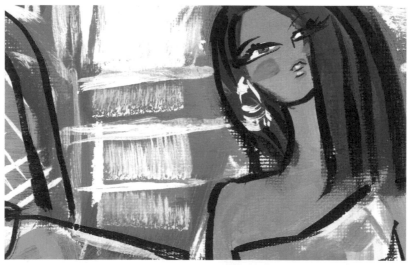

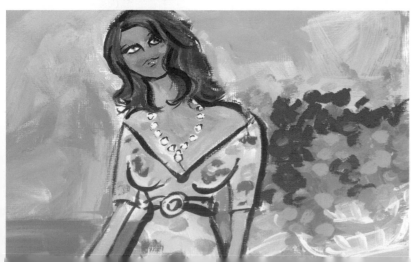

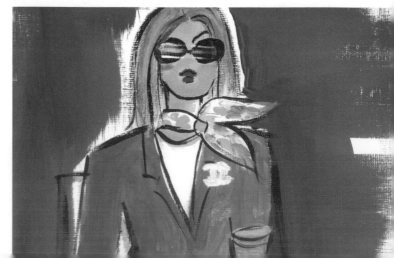

# CHAPTER 4
## Which Archetypal Personality Are You?

An archetype is a symbolic character that represents widely recognized and understood patterns of human nature. It embodies symbols that evoke deep and sometimes unconscious responses. An archetype represents characters, images, and themes that symbolically communicate universal meanings and basic human experiences and consciousness.

I have created seven archetypes that personify unique and universally known attributes that define who women are in the world today. Each expresses her own thoughts, beliefs, emotions, and cultural overlays and dispositions. For those who believe in karma, an archetype expresses "how she came in." Each woman is described by her Defining Qualities, Life Mission and Vision, and Authentic Style Language.

Read through the personalities and identity which archetype best describes your authentic self and conveys your core values, life's work, passions, personal priorities, social preferences, and cultural history. These descriptions will help to demystify and detail your essence and sacred truths. You may find that you have two archetypes. This is not uncommon. The most important aspect of this section is for you to truly discover the soul, spirit, and manifestation of the archetype that defines you so that as you move forward in this book, toward your full expression in dressing and being, you will have a solid foundation to build upon and refer back to for support and connection.

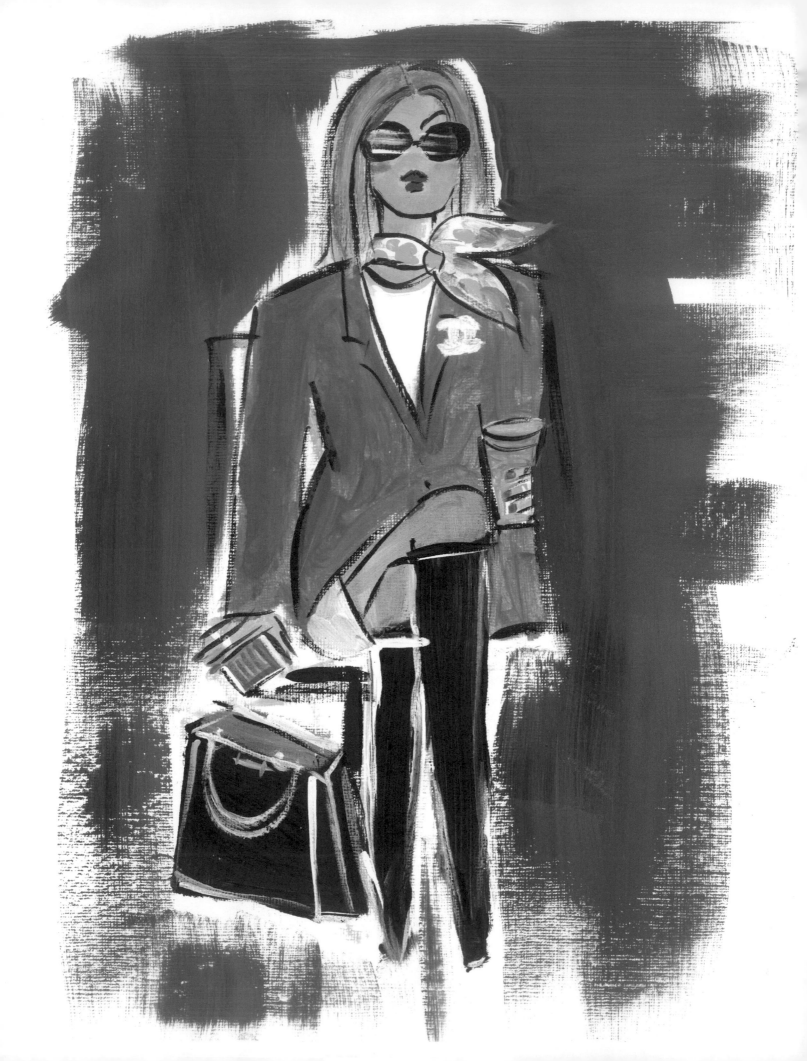

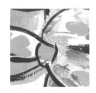

# CHAPTER 5
## The Maverick

### Overview

The Maverick's most extraordinary quality is her will to live fully as herself. She proudly proclaims exactly who she is, what she wants, and how, when and where she is going to manifest her vision. She makes an irrefutable case for why her grand plan is "globally" necessary, and above all, she instinctively knows that her vision will catalyze the world in such a way, that it will be forever changed for the betterment of mankind. This powerhouse is self-possessed, radically self-responsible, and wholly invested in her dream come true. She has a keen sense of self-awareness and an insight into people, places, situations, and opportunities that present themselves to her daily, like cookies on the tray. The Maverick is a big personality. She is passionate, almost fierce in her convictions.

### Defining Qualities and Career Focus

The Maverick is a mighty contender. She plays to win, sharing her wealth with her team, her friends, her family, and her community. Bright, articulate, rebellious, ingenious, impatient, and charismatic, she is a force of nature. The Maverick can be an introvert or an extrovert; sometimes she is both, simultaneously. She is loyal, powerful, hardworking, and exacting. She models excellence and requires it from others. Decisive and all-consuming, she doesn't breathe in all the oxygen in the room...she is all the oxygen in any room that she occupies.

The Maverick has strategy and skill. At times her intensity is hilarious, almost comical. She is paradoxical: impervious and excruciatingly vulnerable. The Maverick can be CEO, chairman, entrepreneur, or a thought leader in her field whether it be an aerospace engineer, fashion designer, philanthropist, corporate iconoclast, surgeon, or five-star chef. She is the driver behind her book of business. She will leave the world a better place...and someone else can see to the details and clean up the leftovers. Her

> *"She has come here*
> *with a vision and a strategy*
> *that is all her own.*
> *This vision will birth a gift*
> *to the world that is*
> *like no other."*

legacy is her life's work. She has celebrity status.

Not all Mavericks seek world domination. They can be PTA presidents and small business owners too. Mavericks rise to the pinnacle of success. The height of her ladder is determined by many things. Her drive, not her circumstances, dictates her success.

## Mission and Vision

She has come here with a vision and a strategy that is all her own. This vision will birth a gift to the world that is like no other. It will leave a legacy for future generations and create a new paradigm, a new perspective, a new totally immersive experience and zeitgeist.... Why is she doing it? Because it needs to be done. How is she doing it? With every fiber of her being. What is her inner motivation? It is a calling that requires total devotion. It is a jealous lover. She was born to do this.

## Style Language

A Maverick's wardrobe must support her mission statement and never compete with her inner brilliance. Her style is dramatic, singular; strong colors and lines, juxtaposed perspectives, decisive form. Functional and fashionable but not trendy. Body conscious but not overly sexy. Garments must command the room as she does, but never eclipse her persona. The Maverick sometimes chooses to create almost a blank slate for herself, so that she can adorn it as her mood and mission suggests. She invests in key pieces that express her exuberance and uniqueness. The underpinnings might be quite retiring and barely there. Quality and craftsmanship are key. Fit and functionality are priorities.

She has no need to wear labels... she is the only label you need to recognize. Perfectly coiffed and perfectly appointed, the Maverick is always appropriately startling. Outlandish or ultraconservative, she makes an entrance, commands the room, and is incredibly keen, perceptive, and inquisitive. Her garments are strategic. They serve as her weapons and her camouflage. Everything about a Maverick is planned and predetermined to achieve her goals. Even her lipstick case has an M.O. Her strategy is platinum. She is not into excess, and she tolerates no competition... especially not her wardrobe.

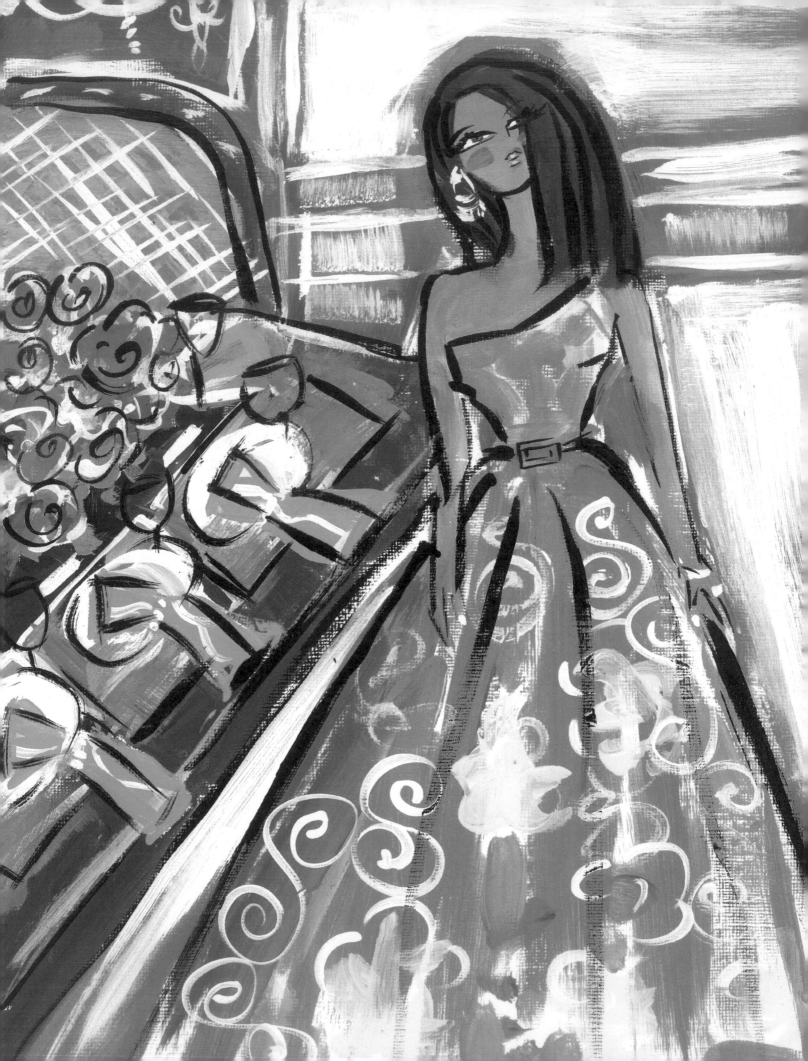

# CHAPTER 6
## The Icon

### Overview

Grace and beauty personified... that is what an Icon is made of. Elegance and poise, gentility and cordiality... kindness and courage... discernment and discretion. The Icon soul possesses a certain transcendent quality that leaves one breathless and refreshed. She glistens with an otherworldly glow...and is remembered and revered long after the party is over. She emanates light and love. She adheres to the rules of decorum and minds her manners in all areas of life. Although she is more than capable of becoming the star of any show, she often prefers to be the supporting role in life's play.

### Defining Qualities and Career Focus

Icons are extraordinary: intelligent, loyal, tactful, silently strong, painfully courteous, and pretty much always right. She has no need to flaunt it... what she's got is ageless, timeless, and pedigreed. Everyone admires this classic woman. She is who we all wish to be. She attends every basketball and track meet rooting from the sidelines, makes costumes for the school play, and raises money for charitable causes. She bakes cookies, delivers dinners, writes notes, and entertains with the utmost style and panache. Miss Etiquette has nothing on the Icon. She is educated, fashion forward, pop culture fluent, and self-effacing and has the patience of a saint. She is born with a clear understanding of her station in life and the responsibilities that come with the designation. She spends her lifetime fulfilling the legacy passed down to her from generations past.

She always does the right thing. She can do almost everything well, standing proudly behind her partner and children. They are her works of art. The Icon is very involved in philanthropy on many levels, making a marvelous board member, worker bee, and hostess. She is a socialite with diplomacy and humility. She tends to shy away from corporate careers as her first priority is family, then community. Occasionally an Icon pierces the veil and becomes an actress, writer, photographer, or model. Or she may elect to be a teacher, therapist, docent, or curator. She can be whatever she wants to be. She is sugar and spice, everything nice, and is a dream walking too!

## Mission and Vision

The Icon dedicates her life in service to her family, friends, and causes. Her vision and mission are to create a compassionate and gentler world beginning in their own home. She is secure in her gifts and talents and is committed to supporting the creation and success of others.

## Style Language

The Icon's style is classic. She prefers lush, high-quality fabrics, delicate colors with an occasional dip into black and red, simplicity, fine lines, and substance. There is nothing trite or faddish about an Icon. She is powerful in her quiet nature. Her wardrobe extends an olive branch to the world as a breath of fresh air, a soft spot to land an ever-anxious glance, and a delight to behold. She prefers to be at home with family and a few close friends. She is always well dressed, her makeup is done right, and her hair is perfectly placed, even when going to the grocery store. She has no need to wear a Statement Maker or try to make an entrance. She is the statement. The room notices her elegant carriage and quiet, exquisite nature. The Icon's perfectly appointed wardrobe is just the bow on the gift of her presence.

*"She can be whatever she wants to be. She is sugar and spice, everything nice, and is a dream walking too!"*

*Grace and beauty personified...*
*that is what an Icon is made of...*
*Elegance and poise,*
*gentility and cordiality...*
*kindness and courage...*
*discernment and discretion.*

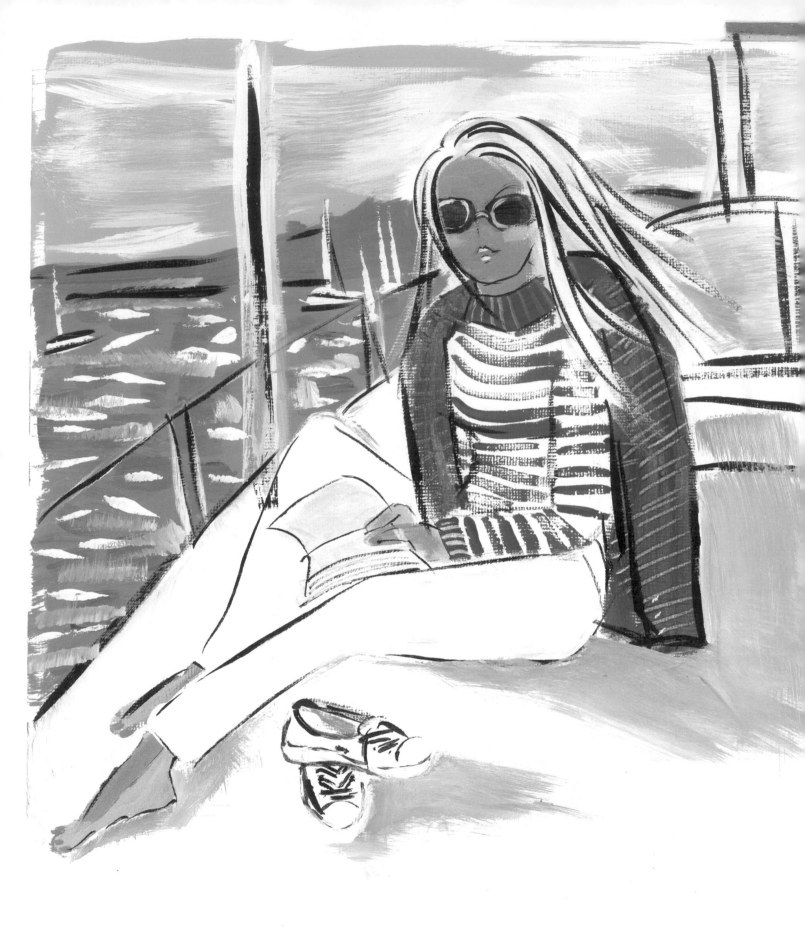

# CHAPTER 7
## The Angelic

### Overview

The Angelic is an angel on earth. Her compassion and kindness are a beacon of light and a shelter for all who need nurturing, protection, and care.

### Defining Qualities and Career Focus

Angelics are the world's healers, advocates, and caregivers who live in service to others as nurturers, humanitarians, teachers, healthcare professionals, volunteers, environmentalists, advocates, and moms. Selfless, nurturing, tender to the core, practical and pragmatic, friendly, and organized; her true north dictates her personal path to self-actualization. She most often works tirelessly with little notice and acclaim. She excels at working in a support role where no one is watching and sharing her talents in an altruistic and very personal way.

### Mission and Vision

The Angelic woman's life mission is to heal the world one soul at a time.

The Angelics come in all shapes and sizes—introverts, extroverts, and everything in between—developing a coping strategy that often masks and protects their ultra-soft center. This barrier allows her to thrive in less than holy environments and maintain her peace of mind while rushing in where angels fear to tread. Sometimes, an Angelic develops an alter ego so that she can accomplish professional goals and personal missions without too much personal exposure. She selects a career that brings joy, satisfaction, and self-worth. She rarely cares about getting credit. An Angelic can be selfless to her own detriment. She is passionate about doing the work that needs to be done, doing it well, and with all her might.

*The Angelic woman is an angel on earth. Her compassion and kindness are a beacon of light and a shelter for all who need nurturing, protection, and care.*

## Style Language

An Angelic's personal style is not flashy, trendy, or cutting edge. She is an action-based girl and extremely practical about her "uniforms." Clothing must be comfortable, functional, and durable. She spends her days in the trenches and needs to wear things that can survive her lifestyle at work and pass as attractive at play. She may never win "Best Dressed" but she always looks nice. She loves casual, easy-to-wear pieces of natural fabrics: cotton, linen, knits, stretchy, skirts, and jeans. She often opts for pants and tops, sweaters and jackets, dresses with pockets, Miss Sincere shoes as well as sneakers and sandals.

Often times, Angelics actually do wear uniforms at work, from scrubs to aprons, or they create their own uniform to save time, money, and overthinking. Angelics like to order clothes online and in department stores. Shopping may not be her favorite pastime, but she appreciates the need to look the part and plays along in order to accomplish her mission. It's not what she wears that makes her day but what she does that brings a smile to her face.

*The Angelic woman's
life mission
is to heal the world
one soul at a time.*

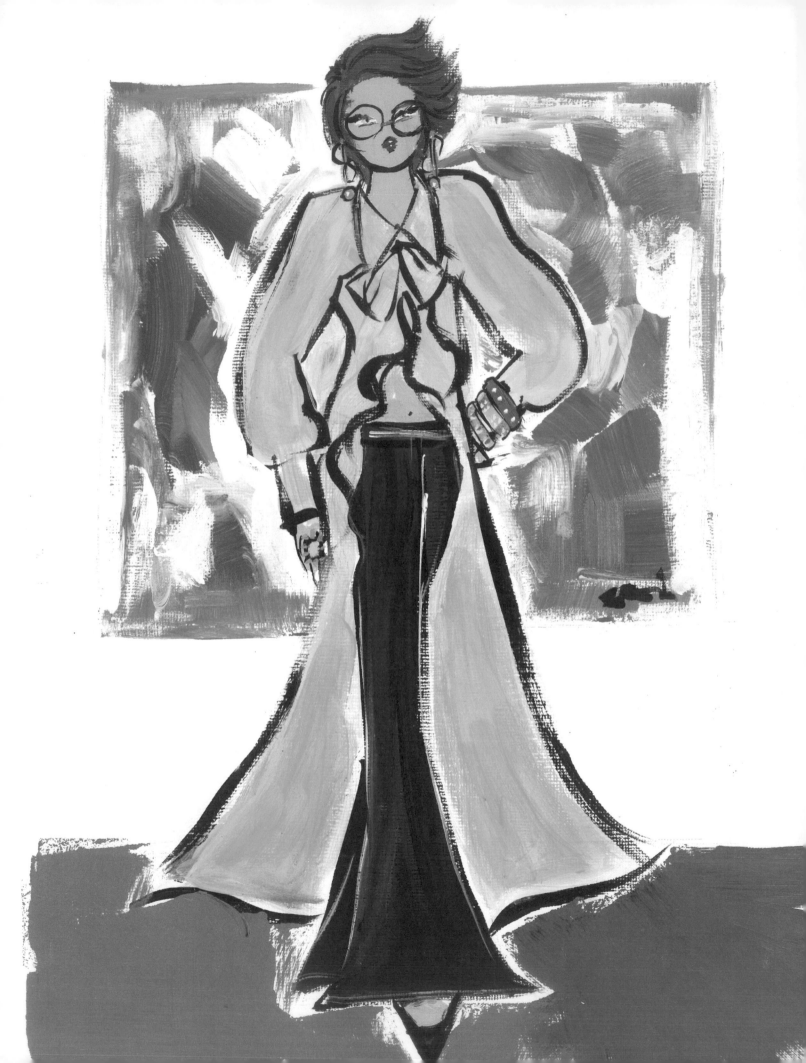

# CHAPTER 8

## The Creative

### Overview

The Creative makes something from nothingness with enthusiasm and exactness. She receives inspiration in direct downloads, vesselling enormous emotion and passion until it can no longer be contained: then art is born. She aspires to embrace, encompass, explore, and awaken life within each of us. A Creative's mission is to make us feel something and take action through the epiphany of her art. The Creative's understanding is entirely unique to her sensibilities, often imitated but never replaced.

### Defining Qualities and Career Focus

The Creative vision is born, not made. She does not choose her destiny. It chooses her. Karma...you know what they say. It's a life sentence. Her life calling, her propulsion and obsession is to birth her vision into the world. Creatives can be obsessed, depressed, impressed, and repressed...but never possessed by anything except the desire to get out of themselves what the divine sewed into them. She is the storyteller and playwright for life's journey, describing the human condition in all forms... deeply knowing the divine comedy of life, expressing each facet of human nature in her unique voice.

A Creative's mission is to create art that changes people's ideas, feelings, and experiences. Her efforts trans-mutate reality into a full immersion sensory experience that describes life's intangible awareness. Creatives are poets and painters, designers and dramatists, composers and actor, artisans and authors, chefs and creative directors, bakers and bohemians, musicians and magicians. Creatives are the imagineers of humankind. They are enthusiasts, sensualists, performers, self-expressionists, and individualists who courageously impose order from chaos, offering it up on an altar of vulnerability and boldness. These unique women are sometimes shy and reclusive; others are brash and arrogant; still others are playful, generous, extroverted, and excitable. No two Creatives are alike.

## Mission and Vision

That which comes through her is far greater than that which comes from her. Creativity is loaned, not owned, and her life is the fleshing out of all that she is given to do. Her art is her obsession, greatest joy, and greatest anguish. This talent is such a gift. Its stewardship is her commitment to her creator and happiness is her reward, when she sees others make her art their own. The Creative woman is in love with the process of channeling the universe. For her own sanity and preservation, she becomes unattached to the result.

## Style Language

The Creative's style sense spans the universe. Some Creatives wear their art like a mantle. Each outfit becomes an extension of her palette. She is her own muse, inhabiting canvases for a monologue, soliloquy to self, and testimony to others. Other Creative women choose to appear as a blank space, allowing their art to be introduced without the hindrance of personality. She chooses to wear a self-created uniform, a monochromatic silhouette, an easel or blank wall to place her masterpieces upon. Some creatives are totally self-conscious and aware of their physical bodies, celebrating their flamboyance and highly personal point of view. Others show up totally "out of their body" and cannot even be bothered to brush their hair or find a clean frock.

Some Creatives find their personal form does not match up to the vision they have for personal expression in fashion. They discard the notion of communicating through their own physical being and focus their creative fashion inspiration on a discovered nymph, a muse, a surrogate self. When this happens, they find a willing being who can fully express their vision of physical beauty. This muse becomes their confidante, inhabiting the vision they have for themselves but are unable to embody.

*"The Creative's
style sense spans
the universe.
Some Creatives wear
their art
like a mantle.
Each outfit becomes
an extension
of her palette."*

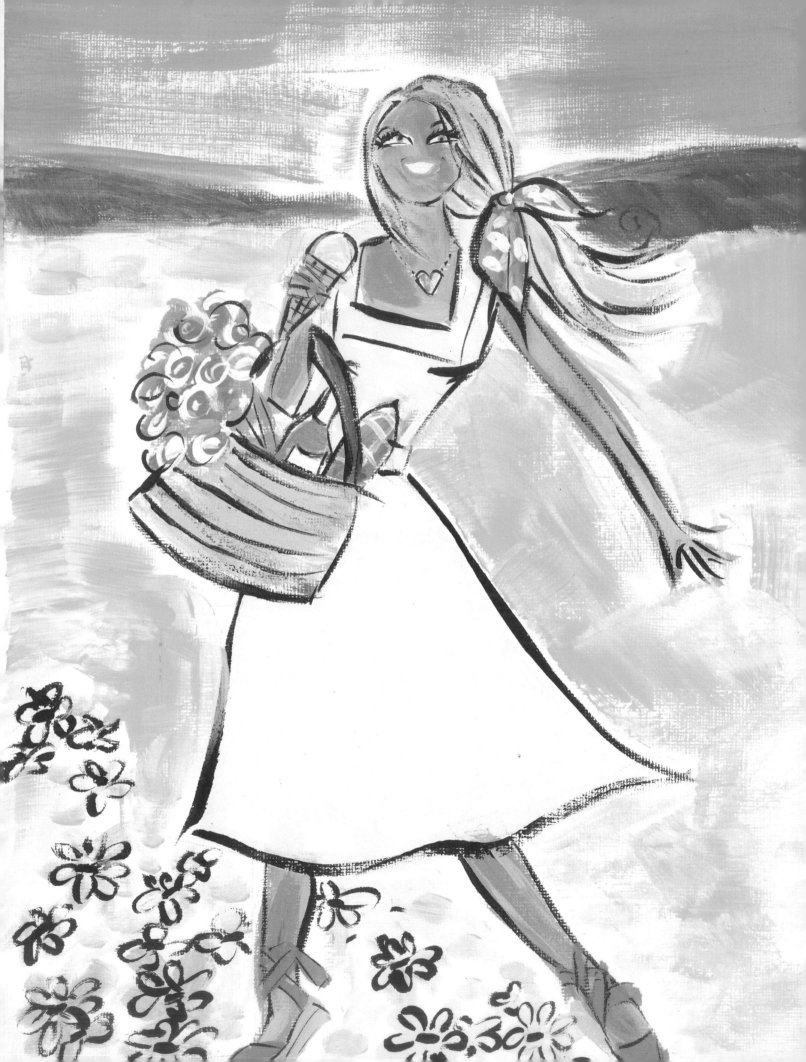

# CHAPTER 9
## *The Innocent*

### Overview

The Innocent is an idealist who emotes vulnerability and naïveté regardless of her age, wisdom, circumstance, and status. Her joie de vivre and passion for purity and joy reaches far beyond any other singular core value. The glass is always full and rosy. She is Holly Golightly, Pollyanna, and the Unsinkable Molly Brown all wrapped into one marvelous being.

### Defining Qualities and Career Focus

The Innocent is resolute about the Utopia she hopes for the world and everyone in it! She is optimistic, whimsical, resourceful, and undaunting in her character. She is courageous and kind. Many fairy tale heroines and romantic leading ladies possess this light, true grit, and intuitive inner voice. Valorous, honest, trustworthy, self-reliant, and intelligent beyond her years; she may begin her journey appearing to be a damsel in distress but becomes the benevolent heroine by the story's end! The Innocent can be found flourishing in many different careers and causes, from nanny to princess and everything in between.

The common denominators for all the Innocents are righteousness, a solid work ethic, and a big cheer for the underdog. She can be involved in charitable causes as a come-hither CEO or flourish as a grassroots volunteer. She often elects to spend her life and career working with children, staunchly advocating on their behalf. Many successful self-made women share this personality and are known for their bravery under fire, whether they become businesswomen, entrepreneurs, corporate executives, or executive directors.

## Mission and Vision

The Innocent's mission is to spread sunshine wherever she goes and bring a bag full of miracles and happiness to share with all in need. She believes in goodness and fairness. The Innocent believes in possibility and is indefatigable in her quest for truth, justice, kindness, generosity, and freedom to be who and what she likes. She is childlike in her approach to life and spunky and precocious in her drive to accomplish her goals in spite of circumstances. She refuses to grow up, give in, or let go of her mission to live life as one big happy sitcom...she heralds her balloons and big top euphoria to all who experience her. The Innocent can be glitter and confetti, grit and girlishness, tomboy and tenacity, or bashful and blushing.... One thing is for sure, once the Innocent enters your life, you will start believing in The Fairy Godmother, Santa Claus, unicorns, and world peace all over again.

## Style Language

The Innocent style is very youthful, light, and airy. She can be ultra-feminine or casual and carefree. Her happy-go-lucky persona is best suited for an Ingenue Muse wardrobe. Nothing too restricted or grown up for this girl. Her wardrobe is a harbinger for her essential persona: light, love, joy, happiness, and pixie dust. She transforms the world with a glance, a prayer, and some pansies. She appears uncomplicated, but deep within her is iron conviction and a clear and utter faith that the world is the ultimate good and so is everyone and everything in it! She is tenacious and true blue in coquetterie: blue jeans, pinafores, organza, or gingham. You can depend on her. She is fearless in her faith, practical, and pretty in her demeanor and guided by a strong conviction for doing what is right.

*"The Innocent style is very youthful, light, and airy. She can be ultra-feminine or casual and carefree. Her happy-go-lucky persona is best suited for an Ingenue Muse wardrobe."*

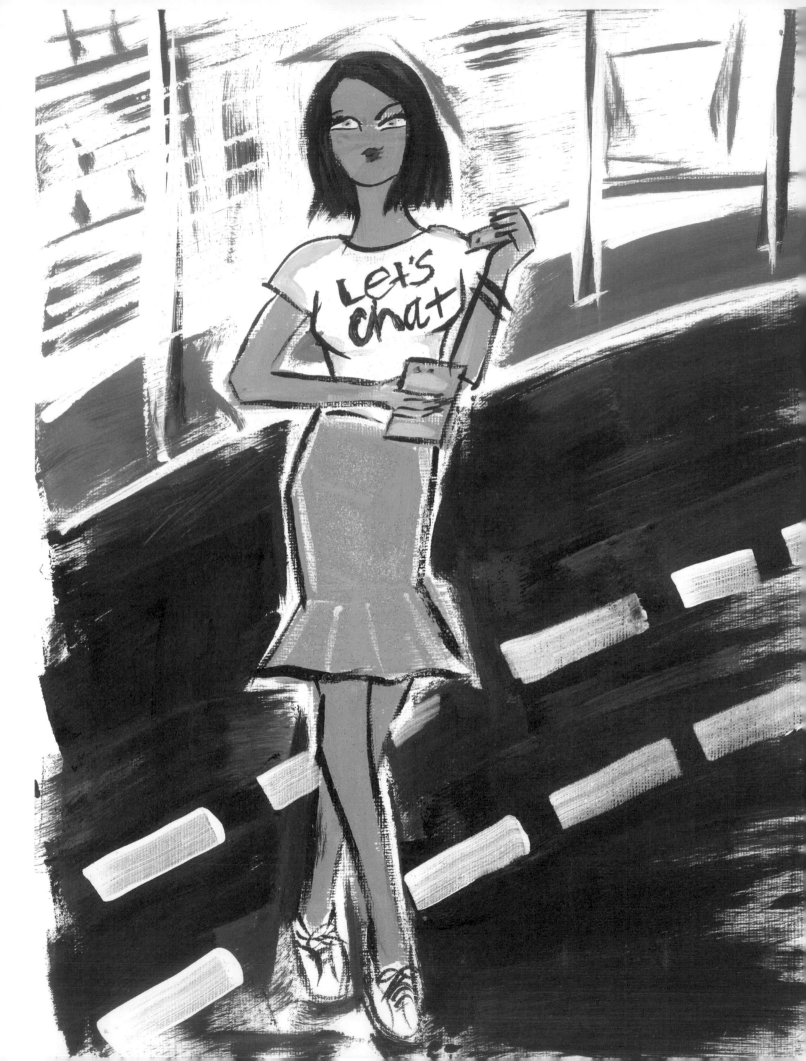

# CHAPTER 10
## The Alchemist

### Overview

The Alchemist is truly defined but not confined by her title. As the chameleon or shapeshifter archetype, this wide-ranging, transmuting being can truly become anything she wants or needs to be to successfully communicate thoughts, share feelings, hold space, educate, emulate, and edify another being. She consumes obtuse knowledge and paradigm-shifting wisdom like fine Champagne, translates it into bite-size, delectable morsels, and offers it up on a silver tray for people to enjoy and digest! She possesses the uncanny ability to communicate large concepts, intangible assets, and huge karmic downloads to any audience in their native tongue and come across being relatable and relevant, all the while knowing her next mission is on its way. Her career options are as vast as her many faces. Her access to the heart, mind, and soul of others sets a new precedent for communication effectiveness and soft-skillset acquisition.

### Defining Qualities and Career Focus

In a very real and palpable way, an Alchemist catalyzes measurable shifts in a person's being whether the transformations are physical, mental, spiritual, or heart-centered. The Alchemist woman sees the world from a totally unique perspective and is able to bring disparate parts together in a holy union that eclipses the success of anything occurring separately. An Alchemist's genius lies in her innate understanding of matter, time, space, emotions, divinity, and intuitiveness. She finds solutions, healing, expertise, and peace in seemingly hopeless and often hapless situations. Her gifts of perception and clarity align with her intelligence, resourcefulness, and extraordinary people skills. She expertly transforms a situation, a person, and opportunity from ordinary to extraordinary. They are problem solvers on a quantum level.

The Alchemist is a catalyst. She is a present-day truth seeker, sorcerous cum spiritualist, enchantress, sage, and illusionist, drawing upon her connection with spirituality coupled with a keen instinctual awareness of human nature. Combine this with extraordinary intuition, amazing timing, and expertise! How do these extraordinary women show up in the world? They are experts, empaths, epigeneticists, light workers, doctors, healers, psychoanalysts, and transformationalists. They are also PR and marketing directors, fundraisers, AI gurus, personal development specialists, attorneys, coaches, and sales professionals, yoginis, and personal trainers. They can be real estate brokers, yacht saleswomen, financial planners, teachers, faith leaders... magicians, visionaries, warriors, and sages.

## Mission and Vision

She is  here to transform the world one by one or thousands by thousands. Her gift is the ability to transform or create something through a seemingly magical process, taking something ordinary and "miraculously" turning it into something extraordinary, sometimes in a way that cannot be explained. An example of using alchemy is a person who takes a pile of scrap metal and turns it into beautiful art. She relies upon her awareness and spiritual connection to Source. Call it God, the Universe, Nature, or Divine Intellect. She connects others to solutions for unsolvable problems and offers ways for people to rise valiantly above their circumstances and triumph in their calling.

## Style Language

The Alchemist has a wardrobe that suits every possible occasion and has outfits to seamlessly establish rapport for every personality along the way. Her closet is like peeking into Central Casting. She transforms her image to best communicate the information she brings to bear, and she leverages every ounce of her being to become the one person in the world who can deliver a message to a specific audience with confidence, clarity, and compassion in the most affable, self-deprecating, and humorous manner. She can also deliver her message with power and panache.... Whenever duty calls, this warrior woman puts on her face paint and feathers and takes the world by storm!

*She possesses the uncanny ability to communicate large concepts, intangible assets, and huge karmic downloads to any audience in their native tongue and come across being relatable and relevant, all the while knowing her next mission is on its way.*

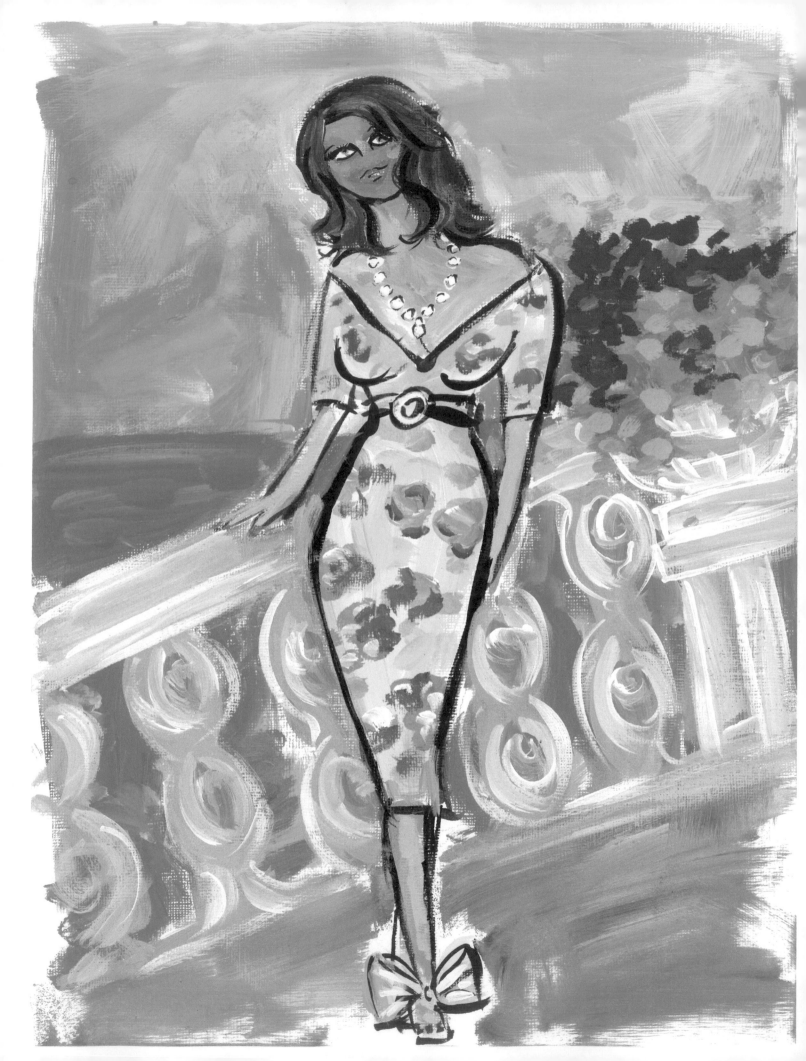

# CHAPTER 11
## The Lover

### Overview

The Lover is also an idealist, and a sensualist... she sees each glass full, participates in every moment with all her might. The Lover is a romantic at heart, tender and naive, sassy and saucy, brave in her utter femininity and generous with her heart, her belongings, and her world. The Lover is usually traditional in her upbringing and an optimist in her worldview. She possesses a certain charisma that leaves a perfume of joy and beauty wherever she goes. She is passionate in her desire to create a beautiful life for herself and her loved ones. She tends to like embellishments and frills using little restraint when it comes to all things floral, ruffles, lace, and sparkles. She is soft, vulnerable, and easily hurt, but beware there is steel behind those magnolias and a resiliency that keeps her youthful and pliable regardless of the years and journey.

### Defining Qualities and Career Focus

The Lover has so many attributes, gifts, and talents. She can be anyone she chooses. Since love is her central focus, she tends to select professions that allow for a full expression of beauty in her life. She is a devoted mother, wife, daughter, sister, friend, and community member. She loves to entertain and be entertained. She loves her home, investing time, energy, and talent into creating gorgeous spaces, places, and objects that convey the gentle life she aspires to live to the fullest.

She has a refined palette, investing and relishing in sensory desires...scents, tastes, touches, sounds, and sights. She is a beauty enthusiast and advocate who spends hours and resources creating and enjoying beautiful homes, parties, wardrobes, experiences, events, and things. Every small detail has been pre-decided, planned, and executed with love, great care, and a discerning eye. She loves luxury and invests in quality.

*The Lover is also an idealist, and a sensualist... she sees each glass full, participates in every moment with all her might. The Lover is a romantic at heart, tender and naive, sassy and saucy, brave in her utter femininity and generous with her heart, her belongings, and her world.*

The Lover is a hopeless romantic in relationships and perspectives, always falling for the prince, hero, or even the jester.

Interior designers, entertainers, teachers, writers, chefs, actors…anything she touches instantly blossoms and grows. She is sometimes unrealistic in her expectations. Her rose-colored glasses are firmly planted and she sees the world through the lens of a beautiful soft-focus movie.

## Mission Statement and Vision

If asked, "What did I come here to do?" she would instantly reply, "I do love." The Lover infuses the world with goodness, optimism, faith, and enthusiasm. She brushes off the dust of everyday life and replaces it with kindness, beauty, and joy. The Lover also creates legacy moments, believing passionately that the past is worth remembering and celebrating. She feels that history informs the present and future in a thoughtful and significant way. A Lover believes that connecting to personal, familial history, and many cultural historic overlays has value for present and future generations, offering roots to give stability and wings to fly. She is well grounded, sentimental, and nostalgic. She designs and curates cameo moments so that everyone can personally embrace and fully understand their personal life journey and relationships along the way.

## Style Language

The Lover adores travel, the arts, fine cooking and wine, architecture, and design… anything sensual in nature. Her style preferences involve luxe fabrics and quality craftsmanship, embellishments, and highly ornate pieces as well as satins, lace, velvets, pearls, baubles, and bows. The Lover's style is alluring and sexy in a femme fatale, ultra-feminine fitted and soft way. She wears her heart on her sleeve, quite literally, and looks fabulous in retro and vintage pieces, accents, proportions, and lines, naturally attracted to rich colors and feel-good fabrics.

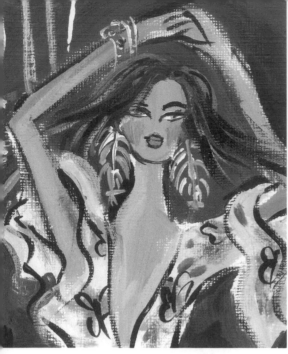

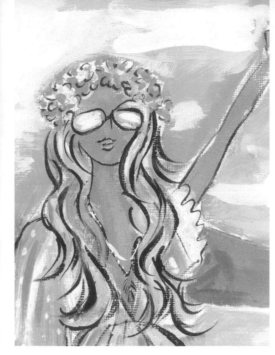

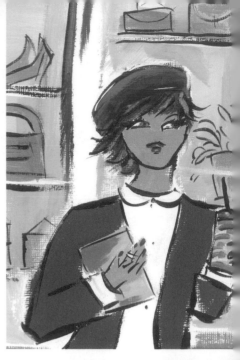

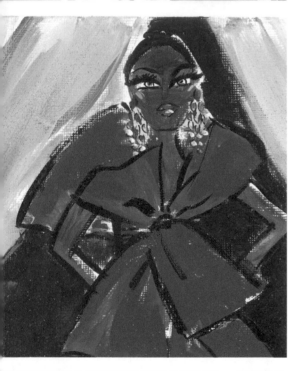

*Style can be defined as beingness. It is the manner of expressing something in behavior, thought, and action.*

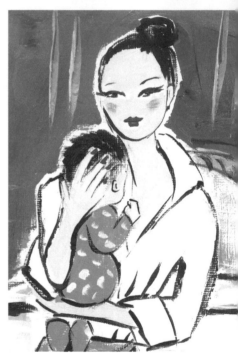

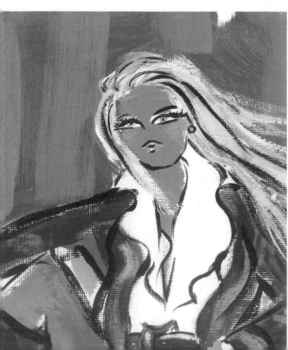

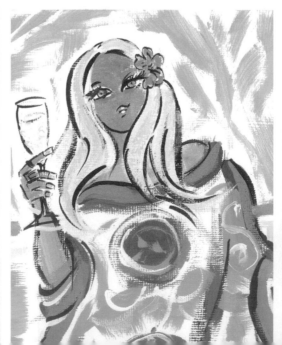

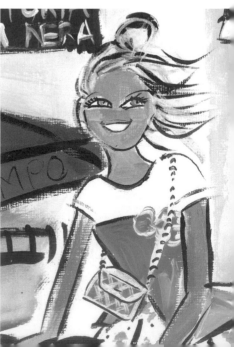

# CHAPTER 12

## What Is Your Style Persona?

Your archetypal personality is your internal truth. It speaks to what you know deeply within your heart and soul about your nature and how you express yourself, interpret reality, and relate to yourself and others. Now that you have a defined understanding of who you are on the inside, it is time to define who you want to see reflecting your authentic self on the outside.

Style is a very personal exploration into the language of self-expression in every area of your life—communication, decorating, entertaining, taste preferences in cuisine, the arts, travel, language, lifestyle, and clothing. Style can be defined as beingness. It is the manner of expressing something in behavior, thought, and action. In fashion, style is a unique way of expressing yourself through clothing.

This chapter will assist you in defining your personal style in clothing and lifestyle. The two really cannot be separated. We spend time in clothes that serve a specific purpose. We dress according to the tasks at hand. The focus of this chapter is to help you apply what you see on the runway to you. It will assist you in creating what feels good and clearly expresses who you are each day. Clothes are decorative for certain; they are also very functional. It's imperative that when you walk into your closet every morning that you find something to wear for the many roles you play each day. It is crucial that you feel like yourself. It is paramount that your second skin portrays you for who you truly are... not who you would like to be in a virtual world. You must not only like what you wear, you must be able to navigate your day in what you wear. Your lifestyle has a lot to do with your choices, and your schedules and commitments have a lot to do with what will work for you and not against as you celebrate your everyday self in fashion.

I have created eight style personas: The Entrance Maker, The Eternal Beauty, The Hopeful Romantic, The Bohemian Rhapsody, The Explorer Naturalist, The Carefree Casual, The Ingenue Muse, and The Energetic Sprite. Each persona is defined by her spiritual presence, style language, and wardrobe style. We go on to explore her as an earthly being and see her point of view through the eyes of society. After reading through each persona, select the one or two that feel like you, supports your lifestyle, and embodies your fashion sense. This is your style persona.

*Style is a very personal exploration into the language of self-expression in every area of your life—communication, decorating, entertaining, taste preferences in cuisine, the arts, travel, language, lifestyle, and clothing.*

*Clothes are decorative for certain;*
*they are also very functional.*
*It's imperative that when you*
*walk into your closet every morning*
*that you find something to wear*
*for the many roles you play*
*each day.*

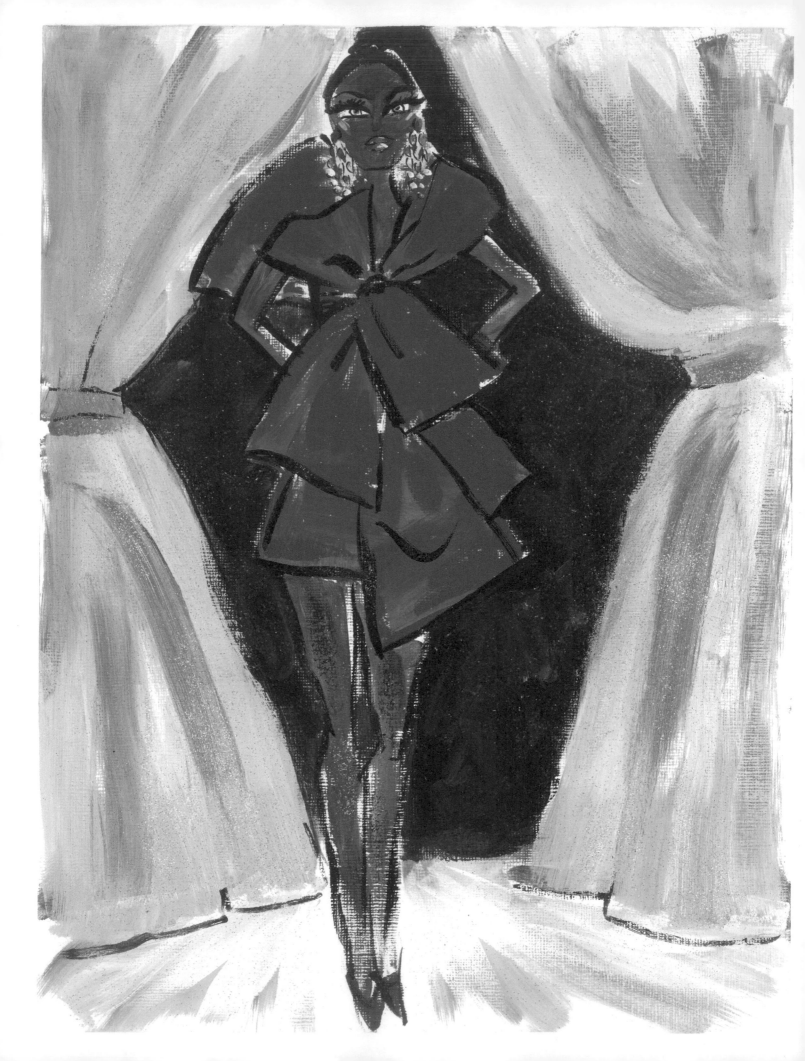

# CHAPTER 13
## The Entrance Maker

The Entrance Maker is dramatic and intentional in her personality and her style, counting on her visage to launch ships, move mountains, and sing the "Hallelujah" chorus at the drop of a hat. She is a self-proclaimed prophet and her clothes are part of an elaborate scheme for world domination and prestige. There are no accidents in an Entrance Maker's wardrobe or lifestyle. Every piece has a purpose and she wears each well. Clothing is her ammunition. Ambition is her trajectory, and intimidation, seduction, and power is her game.

Her mission is simple: She was given a birthright responsibility to change the world and create a new paradigm in whatever field she chose. She has enormous strength of character, remarkable physical and mental stamina, and a clear vision for how much improved and upgraded a specific experience and lifestyle will be once her concepts are articulated and manifested under her direction.

She approaches all situations with laser focus. She always gets her way. She is dead set on setting the world ablaze and leverages every hemline, stiletto, and lipstick to achieve her goals. Her uniforms are those of elite warriors, and she has an ensemble for every occasion. Each is perfectly complete to the last accessory. The fit is magnificent. The color is unforgiving, and the style is superhuman. She loves exaggerated lines and flares or absolute minimalism. She can be stealth or steely. Her presence is commanding and awe-inspiring. Her clothes are a tool. Her image chiseled. Her communication intense.

Bombshell or Beauty Girl, Femme d'Affaires or Femme Fatale, the Entrance Maker creates a hush, takes a bow, and leaves no prisoners. She is fierce and fabulous, omniscient and omnipresent, decisive and daring. The Entrance Maker is a top-notch, A-grade pearl and the world is her oyster.

# Visual Grammar

The Entrance Maker personality, a dramatic, is best expressed as a sophisticated and edgy high-fashion look. Some elect to be outrageous in their attire and effect. One thing is for sure, being "over the top" suits their personality just fine. Her entrances are unforgettable and her presence makes waves! Her appearance is modern art, expressionist, obtuse, and surreal. It's film noire meets epic fantasy. She is a walking billboard, bold, trendy, smoldering, or severe.

The more sophisticated Entrance Maker exudes a richer appearance and sensibility, allowing her seamless entry into professional settings and discriminating social circles. She is a head-turner, pleasing her loyal audiences with her colossal presence and poise. She is all mystery, majesty, and inspiration.

The more trendy, artsy, dramatic Entrance Maker chooses to work in creative fields such as fashion, interior design, architecture, and culture. Her fashion choices are dramatic in cut, color, and design. She is a risk-taker who never disappoints with her daring and larger-than-life selections and commentary.

The other visual grammar choice for the Entrance Maker is absolute minimalism with superb extreme tailoring and monochromatic. Her strategy is to create a vacuum instead of an explosion. This drastic imposed uniform is almost militaristic, intending to direct the viewer's eye wherever she chooses. Some Entrance Makers don't want to steal the show, preferring to observe the circus, watch the opera from box seats, and hold court with their inner circle. Fit, fabric, and proportion are key facets in creating this zeitgeist.

# The Earthly Being

**Body Type**
- Height usually tall (5'8" plus) or under 5'5"
- Bone structure narrow & angular or broad & balanced
- Overall look exotic, striking, not classic, or totally "unpretty"—even homely

**Facial Features**
- Chiseled and angular
- Prominent features such as a prominent nose, high cheekbones, or angular jawline based upon DNA or adopted history

**Hairstyle**
- Sleek, geometric, or asymmetrical work best
- Avoid layers and curls or soft shapes

**Makeup**
- Can be all or nothing at all, depending upon the archetype
- Bold lipstick works for some
- Eyelashes and glam for others
- Bare-faced with a hint of color for the more circumspect Entrance Makers

## Wardrobe Style

**Key Elements**
- Hot off the runway look works wonders for the dramatic
- Flamboyant and trendy or severe and minimalist work best
- Statement pieces with accessories
- Ensemble dressing is an everyday staple for this sophisticated entrepreneurial spirit
- "Go-to" pieces are absolutely necessary in an Entrance Maker's wardrobe. Between her busy social calendar and professional life, she has to have certain outfits that are "Wows" every time. They become perennial favorites.
- Strong colors in large patterns and geometrics
- Solids in black, white, red, fuchsia
- Lines should be sleek, long, and straight
- High fashion garments and severely tailored pieces
- Shoulder lines are sharp, angular, or square
- Necklines have angles and edges or occasional scoops or Peter Pan collars.
- Extreme and exotic for evening
- Elongated draping is the only acceptable softness in line; or minimalist and man-tailored suiting

**Fabric**
- Fabrication must be well-defined and hold its shape
- Gabardines, faille, stiff brocades, taffetas, heavy woolen or microfiber knits with structured lines
- Patterns are bold and sweeping, geometric or abstract
- Monochromatic dressing in a single color is sensational
- Color blocking (think Rothko) works as well

**Details**
- Flamboyant, lavish, extreme, and oversized
- Man-tailored or severely tailored are great
- Proportions are large to achieve contrast in silhouette—or extremely close to the body... but not sexy... more androgynous and anonymous

## Unflattering Choices

- Overdoing the look. More is not more here. It actually becomes less.
- Delicate, intricate, and small details do not work
- Flouncy, frilly, and flowing lines
- Anything round, swirling, or too draped
- Overly sheer, lightweight, or extremely rough textures

## Shopping Tips

- If the budget is available, every season is Christmas! If not, buy a minimum amount of well-fitting solid staple pieces and rely upon your accessories to make a splash.
- Purchase neutral classic statement pieces that are interchangeable and seasonless.
- Focus on current trends in clothing and accessories.
- Only buy what is absolutely phenomenal. Fit has to be spot-on or the outfit will not work. Pass on runner-up outfits.
- In budgeting, accessories are key. They complete the look and show off uniqueness and persona. Luxe accessories imbue the sophistication and power of this dynamic personality.
- Ensemble dressing is key to creating a powerful controlled presence.
- Know the labels that are showstoppers and invest in only garments that sets her apart from the rest.

## Accessories

Accessories are statement pieces for the Entrance Maker, worn to evoke an emotion or a thought and catalyze a chain reaction. She prefers oversized singular jewelry pieces to create a center of gravity for her image such as a necklace, brooch, earrings, watch, or ring. She has her favorites. Purses are functional and aesthetically pleasing. They are rarely large after hours, sleek and beautiful over huge and resembling a kitchen sink. Shoes can be utterly utilitarian and clunky or stiletto and razor sharp.

Her clothing is her mantle, chainmail, and shield...it is her weaponry for the battle. She is a warrior. Her wardrobe is her trademark, camouflage, crown and distraction.

Drama is her intention—in words and actions as well as demeanor. She is a take-charge, strong, opinionated influencer. Direct, demanding, and critical, this gal will rule her kingdom and yours. Does she have a soft side? Somewhere. But you will never see her blush. She exists in all walks of life at the top of her field. Entertaining is lavish and

*There are no accidents in an Entrance Maker's wardrobe or lifestyle. Every piece has a purpose and she wears each well. Clothing is her ammunition. Ambition is her trajectory, and intimidation, seduction, and power is her game.*

legendary. Business is fierce and fast moving. She tends to own her own business and be her own boss because all control must reside within her grasp. She is very private about her life and emotionally impenetrable. She does treat people with generosity and grandness and truly has a huge heart hidden somewhere under her aloofness and rapid-fire repartee. The Entrance Maker is unforgettable.

The Entrance Maker can also be seen as making over-the-top fashion choices to the point of almost trashy.... This paparazzi-monopolizing, awe-inspiring, and blood pressure-raising woman does not necessarily care about couture. She cares about creating a Richter-scale-breaking earthquake upon her arrival and is only satisfied if the aftershocks last all night. She may not have a purpose other than being the center of attention. She is somebody. Today everybody can be famous for 15 minutes. So, Snapchat it up, baby...your insta-life is blowing up and you are en fuego!

She is feared and admired. Her clothes are her armor. They don't have to be comfortable; they do have to serve a purpose. Her off-duty wardrobe is still requisite-like fatuous. Only when she retires does her body fully relax into a lush robe, cashmere leggings, plush sweats and slippers. Retiring is just surrender to humanness for the evening so that she can recharge and refresh for tomorrow's battle.

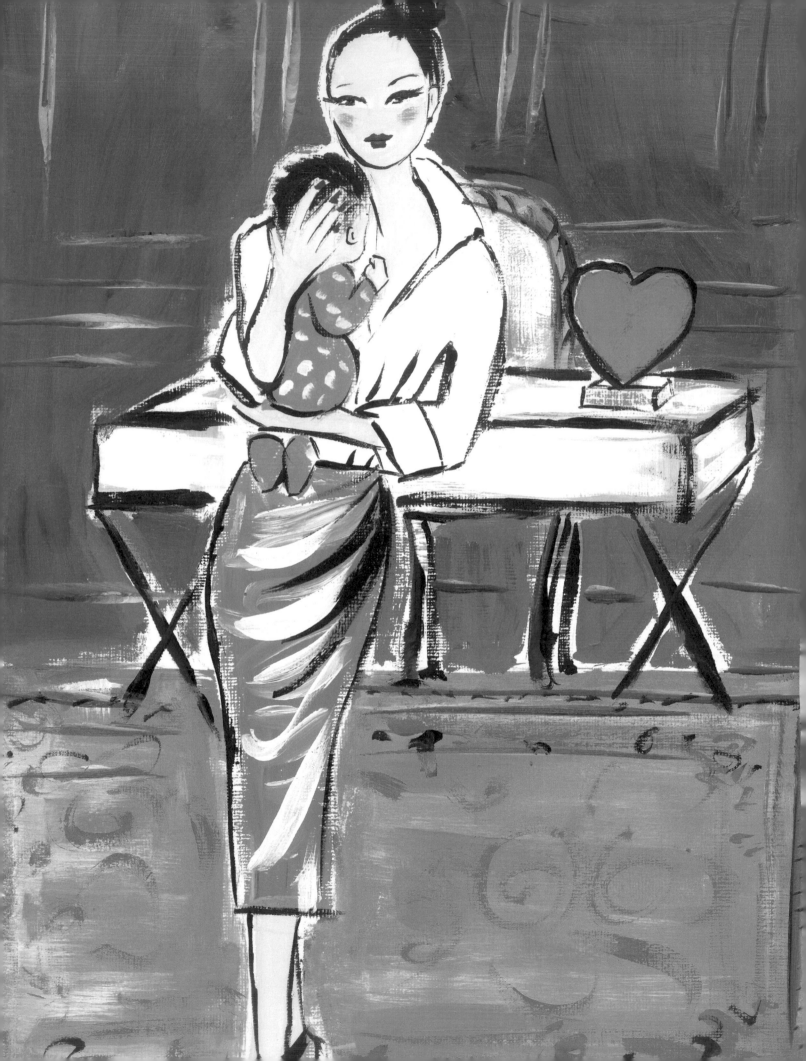

# CHAPTER 14

## *The Eternal Beauty*

The Eternal Beauty is a classic. She is the epitome of elegance, grace, and refinement. Her look is timeless, fashionable, gentle, and luxurious.

## The Spiritual Persona

The key to creating an authentic style for an Eternal Beauty is to embrace her innate destiny... a pedigree beyond wealth, a visceral understanding of what is highest and best, which manifests itself as dignity with purpose. The Eternal Beauty is born with a legacy. Her life purpose maintains and sustains her genteel heritage with all its facets (familial, social, and philanthropic responsibilities) with grace and kindness, courage and decorum.

Her worldview doesn't allow for errors of any kind. She was born to carry out the traditions of her family with honor and translate them elegantly for future generations to embrace and experience. The Eternal Beauty has a very high set of standards. She is a perfectionist at heart. She is taught to play by the rules of the game and understands her part in the intricate puzzle of social status and wealth. She is a loving and loyal wife, a fiercely protective, gently sweet and kind mother, a faithful sister, a dutiful daughter, a forever friend, and a generous humanitarian. She has come to this world to love and support her family and better her community with all her heart and means.

She is an ambassador, an advocate, a fighter for social injustice, a patron of the arts, and a room mother. She is honest, integrous, patient, supportive, moral, and traditional in her values. She admires strength, character, lineage, and subtle charm. She has a great sense of humor and can be charming and attentive. She can also be reserved and retiring, almost hermetic, which can come across as being snobby and aloof. She puts all her energy into her daily routine and needs to take time alone to re-energize, renew, refresh, and restore herself.

She needs time to be alone. She reappears as the gorgeous woman she is known to be. Always measuring up, takes a toll on her...and by the way, she uses the same yardstick for others. She will never arrive anywhere without being dressed and coiffed. Her standards are high and so are her expectations.

## The Visual Grammar

The Eternal Beauty possesses a sense of perfection and clarity. She maintains and expands her sense of discretion and discernment in her wardrobe. This gal is all about a reserved sense of beauty and can be easily made to look clown-like if forced to wear too much of anything. Clean lines and proportion are her friend. Perfect fit and minimal embellishments allow her serene and regal nature to shine. She captures and communicates her essence with high-quality investment pieces in silk, charmeuse, jersey, and fine wools. She loves the crispest voile and linen as well as the drape of cashmere and boucle. She also wears well-manufactured blends that enhance fit and form and do away with those unsightly fabric wrinkles. Her design choices are always classic, and once she determines the designers that express her sensibilities fluently, she tends to stick to that brand for a lifetime.

The Eternal Beauty is timeless. Aging for her is just a number. Her passion for fashion manifests in classic pieces. Appropriateness is key. The Eternal Beauty does have an alluring, sexy side but it is more about showing a little and letting the viewer imagine a lot, looking fabulous in illusion netting or lace, a hint of leg, a sweetheart, portrait, bateau, or strapless neckline. Her clothing reveals the curve of her figure. It's tight enough to show her assets but not so tight as to give away all her secrets. Her wardrobe language is fluent in good manners, proper etiquette, and quiet strength. She does not need to draw attention to herself with her wardrobe. She is instantly recognized.

The Eternal Beauty's style and persona is intentional, controlled, thoughtful, and conservative. She loves to be organized and understated in her words and demeanor. Orderliness and structure at work, at play, and at home give her a sense of freedom and well-being. Her serenity and cool sophistication impose order in any social gathering. A great manager and administrator, she is a diplomat at heart. Her relationships are a social contract of the most refined sort. This classic personality expresses herself heart and soul in her appearance. She reflects the decorated life she enjoys. She is warm and caring, sincere and loyal, faithful, responsible, and trustworthy.

She tends to get "stuck" in her much-loved pieces, which can prematurely age her appearance over time, making her appear matronly and older than her years. At times she appears extremely conservative in her morals, politics, and social mores. It's important for her to step out on the town and keep in touch with current runway looks and fashion styles. Incorporating a few new pieces every season will keep her up to date without being trendy. Makeup and hairstyle are also sticking points. It is so important to update both annually, as wearing the same makeup and hairdo all her life can age her prematurely. Embracing changes and updates will enhance her fabulous face!

## The Earthly Being

- Average height range 5'4" to 5'7", occasionally a bit taller
- Figure evenly balanced, symmetrical
- Overall appearance is ladylike, not girlish
- Body is not too thin or delicate

### Facial Features
- Average to attractive to beautiful
- Symmetrical and well balanced, not long, wide, angular, or round

### Hairstyle
- Shoulder length or slightly longer
- Above the shoulder to chin length
- Neat and controlled
- Blunt cut or smooth, sometimes with layers
- Occasional soft curl
- She often wears longer hair in a neat chignon, French twist, or ponytail

## Wardrobe Style

### Key Elements
- Wardrobe capsule enthusiast
- Fully coordinated from head to toe, including all accessories and jewelry
- Outfit creation instead of mix and match pairings
- Investment dressing
- Basics in solid colors first; florals, patterns, and trends later
- Luxury fabrications
- Excellent tailoring and perfect fit
- Keeps an eye on fashion trends; keeps current but never a fad follower
- Wears what looks best
- Impeccable maintenance and care

# *"Buy less, spend more. Style is eternal... Invest in quality over quantity."*

## Clothing
- Styles are fashionable, dignified, classic, contemporary, and upscale
- Lines are softly tailored and softly flowing, not too body-hugging
- Suiting is "dressmaker" style, not too man-tailored in cut and proportion. Bias is best. Her best lines are neither too straight nor too curvy.
- Trendy, faddish, severe, and overtly sexy is not her style
- Solid colors dominate her palette
- Although she is not a big label wearer, she is a discreet luxury brand wearer and collector
- Loves slacks as much as she loves dresses and suits
- Owns jeans but only her hairdresser knows
- Her casual wardrobes are as equally pulled together as her dressy attire. Even her "at home" attire is perfectly matched.
- She loves sweater sets and pencil skirts, sheath dresses with matching jackets, capris or white jeans with classic blazers
- She is always dressed and ready to receive guests at all times
- Lines are softly flared or straight-refined and smooth
- Proportions are not oversized or exaggerated
- Clean necklines are best kept simple or draped
- Any intricate work such as lace appliqué should be subdued

## Fabrics
- Matte finishes and low lusters are best for key pieces
- Richness and quality are key
- Fabric weights are usually medium
- Layering is lovely but minimal
- Refined textures create a luxe sensibility—silks, woolens, cashmere, gabardines, and crisp cottons
- Smooth knits and double knits are essentials
- Minimal embellishments and shine

## Accessories
- Jewelry, belts, handbags, and shoes are refined, elegant, and fashionable. Again, they are luxurious but not garish.
- Jewelry may be smooth, rounded, geometric, or chunky but they must be classic in nature and eternal in style. There will be no funky dangly ditties for this girl. She tends to have a piece or two that she wears every day and becomes her signature look.

**Unflattering Choices**
- Boring an ultraconservative clothing will appear matronly and staid
- Excessive angles, oversized garments, and severe straight lines
- Fabrics that are too lightweight or too heavy make a classic appear dowdy
- Heavy rough fabrics and weaves, stiff metallics, ultra-sheer, and extremely clingy fabrics
- High-color contrasts and multicolor splashes in prints and patterns
- Poor fit and oversized cuts
- Clothing that lacks shape and is amorphous in nature

**Shopping Tips**
- Plan the budget wisely.
- Invest in the basic wardrobe pieces surrounding a single neutral color choice per season and a contrast color. Buy additional collection pieces on sale. Add an accent color that can change and freshen your look easily.
- "Less is more." Buy quality not quantity.
- Ensemble dressing works best. Complete the look from head to toe. Focus on one ensemble at a time.
- Line, proportion, fit, and fabrication are key to wardrobe success.
- Stay current in the visual language
- Shop on Monday morning and buy on presale.
- Use a stylist or personal shopper who knows one's preferences and what works. Have them pull clothes and dress the room with potential wardrobe pieces, a light lunch, and champagne.

The Eternal Beauty will always be the most revered woman in the room… and her wardrobe often imitated but never truly duplicated. The Eternal Beauty's fashion motto is: "Buy less, spend more. Style is eternal. Be fashionable, not faddish. Invest in quality over quantity." The Eternal Beauty allows her outfit to introduce who she is but never lets it up-stage her authentic self and true nature. She is in a class by yourself.

An Eternal Beauty has a very demanding social schedule requiring quick go-to pieces that are always appropriate and well appointed. She is photo-op ready, fully Instagrammable at every moment, and has amazing memory for what she and everyone else wore to a party years ago. Her closet is as organized as her date book and calendar. Boxes are carefully labeled and arranged seasonally. She is a gracious hostess at home and away from home. She is also a gracious guest—never arriving without a hostess gift… never leaving without a complimentary comment and a follow-up thank you note or call. She is a matriarch at heart. She just allows everyone to think that they are leading the band.

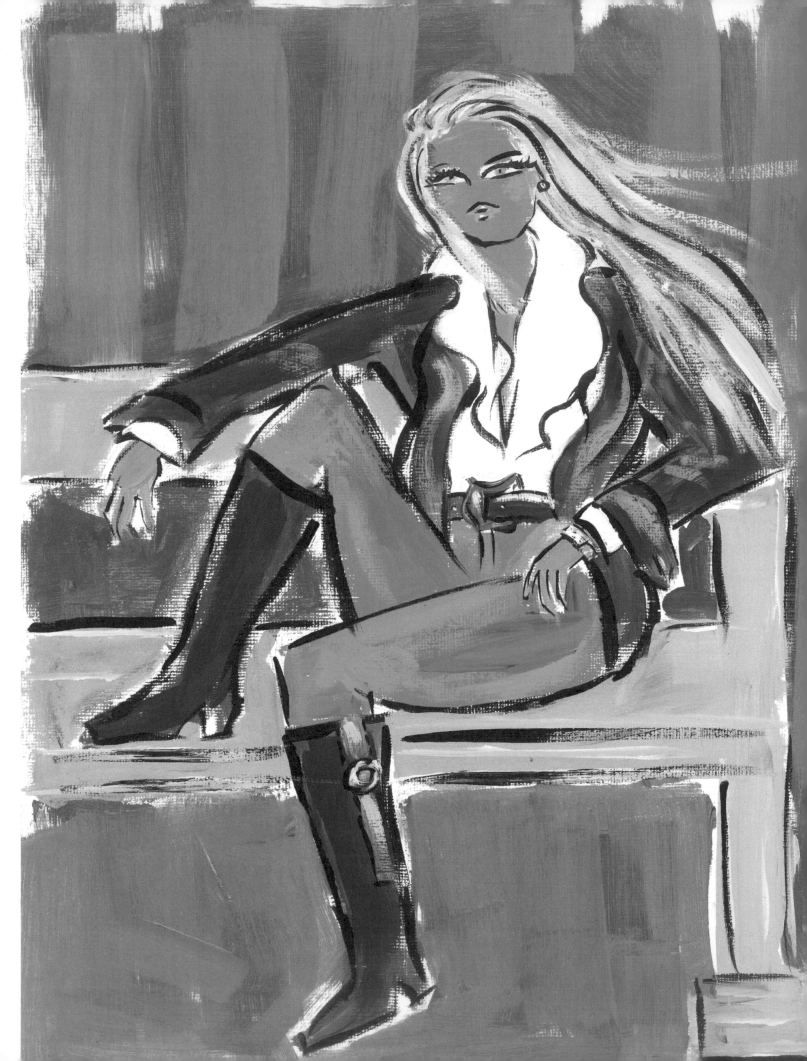

# CHAPTER 15
## *The Explorer Naturalist*

### The Spiritual Persona

The Explorer Naturalist makes her home wherever her soul takes her, loving all things natural and embracing the wanderlust and wonderful spirit of living as one with her surroundings. Whether that be an oceanfront villa in Palm Beach, an all-naturally curated oasis-like loft in NYC, glamping in a national park or living in a suburban Zen garden, one thing is for sure: this beauty relishes bringing all that is beautiful in the outdoors into her home, office, vacation spots, and wardrobe. She delights and insists upon all-natural fabrics, soothing, subtle colors and designs, aroma-infused spaces, and the sound of nature.

The Explorer Naturalist's life mission is to live authentically and honestly and in total respect of our planet and its inhabitants. She is passionate about living in relationship with Mother Earth and spends time and resources protecting our natural world and living in a clean, unhurried, and toxin-free home. She loves animals and wildlife, bonfires, and remote vacations where the device-driven economy and society are silenced and conversations with loved ones are amplified. She is an advocate of slow living, even if her daily schedule is busy and urbane.

If she can't make it from scratch, she will find a way to have it provided for herself and family. Her lifestyle is peaceful and orderly. Her look is very pulled together and easy on the eyes and body. She has a place for everything and everything has a place. If cleanliness is next to Godliness, she lights a daily candle to illuminate her natural sense of order and divinity in everyday life. She is attractive without necessarily being beautiful. Her manners and carriage are confident and easy. She and her body get along very well…. When one speaks, the other listens—a truly symbiotic match.

# Visual Grammar

The Explorer Naturalist always appears as though she is unhurried, present, and confident. She is friendly without being overbearing and practical, consistent and constant in her tastes and style. The Naturalist wardrobe personality embodies the spirit of the All-American woman—manifested in her heart and lifestyle. She is sporty, outdoorsy, patriotic, true blue, and practical in all areas of her life.

Her wardrobe and lifestyle are designed for "ease of use," offering maximum comfort and enjoyment. She is a straightforward woman who knows herself very well and is comfortable and confident about who she is inside and out and the roles she plays in the world. This woman likes to be comfortable at all times. She wants her look to be low maintenance but attractive, just like her personality. She opts for less structured, mix and match garments based upon her favorite wardrobe staples, perhaps her favorite jeans, boots, jacket, or shirt.

She tends to choose professions that enhance her personality—so there is no need for suiting and restrictive garb. Her work wardrobe is synonymous with her daily wear except it's brought up a notch in quality and continuity. For these occasions, the Naturalist will tend to select items from the more classic, Eternal Beauty persona, which suit her body type and sensibility. "Dressing up" can be challenging, but the contemporary form-fitting pieces work well.

The Explorer Naturalist adheres to ensemble dressing. She carefully selects her palette and pieces that work for her daily routine. She then mixes and matches for variety and occasion. Nothing is overdone in this closet. The motto is "function over form." She has the maximum ability to wear sport jackets, skirts, pants, and tops in various colors, textures, and layers and look terrific once the outfit is pulled together. Her persona is youthful, easygoing, approachable, and fashionable but never overdone. Her style conveys that homey, lived-in feeling. Her earthy sensuality gives her a sexiness that is fresh and outdoorsy, no matter what she wears—T-shirts, hiking boots, or just jeans and a white button-down shirt. People are attracted to her natural good looks and pristine outlook.

Think denim. It's a lifelong staple. Think white, crisp, cotton, tailored shirts. Think silk jersey T-shirts and sweater sets. Think cashmere, great-fitting slim slacks, knit pull-ons. She opts for ensembles in beige, taupe, brown, winter white, pearl gray. Her wardrobe must be practical, useful, multi-seasonal, layered, and not flashy. Dresses are more flowy than fitted. She loves blazers and dusters. She is a visual vacation; encountering this gal is like taking a mini staycation. Her presence is calming, relaxing, balanced, and energetically connected. She looks you in the eyes, listens, and smiles, making everyone feel at home and welcome.

Fabric choice is a key decision in her wardrobe. Texture can be varied, including woven and knits to enhance her approachability and individuality. Her accessories are minimal and functional. Her evening attire is a challenge. The solution is to borrow from one of the other personalities that is somewhat aligned with her beliefs and body type. Manufacturers make more evening choices for the Eternal Beauties and Hopeful Romantics. Simpler elegance is the best choice: brocades, crepes, micro-fibers, jerseys, velvets, and channel beading for glamour.

# The Earthly Being

**Body Type**
- Height is average to tall
- Strong and sturdy build, straight or curvy
- Muscular and athletic with a broader shoulder
- Bone structure is softly angular

**Facial Features**
- Shape is broad (round or square) or oblong
- May be asymmetrical with a broadness
- Nose may be broad and flat

**Hairstyle**
- Tousled, loose, windblown, uneven
- Never fussy, always "wash and wear"
- Not too blunt or smooth

# Wardrobe Style

**Key Elements**
- A little bit country, a touch western
- Urban chic with a feminine roughness
- Athletic and easy
- Jeans always and everywhere
- Mix and match
- Easy on the eyes and heart
- Practical, earthy, natural sexiness
- Comfort is key

**Clothing Style**
- The look is upscale backpacker, horse woman, boating enthusiast, skier, photojournalist
- Garments are not overly structured or stiff. Tailoring is simple and soft.
- Lycra added to fabrics for comfort, durability, and appeal
- Not fussy and perfect fit
- Allows for maximum movability—nothing to restricted or plastic wrap tight
- Minimal details
- Separates dominate the wardrobe closet
- Mix and match patterns, textures, and colors
- Designer sportswear is the look

**Fabrics**
- Textures can be soft, rough, or nubby
- Crinkled or wrinkled works fine with the addition of a few starched shirts
- Knits can be jersey, cabled, studded, or nubby
- Raw silks can be wonderful as well as tweeds, flannels, wools, challis, linens, cottons, flannels, cashmeres, leathers, and denims

**Accessories**
- Avoid too many accessories
- Best suited for a great earring and a great watch
- High-quality hats, belts, bags, and shoes
- Boots of all shapes and looks
- Loafers, car shoes and espadrilles
- Pumps
- Structured sandals
- Couture scarves are her favorite addition worn many ways

**Unflattering Choices**
- Severely man-tailored looks that destroy her femininity
- Comfort only. Can look sloppy instead of stylish.
- Grooming is key to a natural look—skin care and a great haircut and/or color is essential

*The Explorer Naturalist's life mission is to live authentically and honestly... She is passionate about living in relationship with Mother Earth and spends time and resources protecting our natural world and living in a clean, unhurried, and toxin-free home.*

## Shopping Tips

- The Explorer Naturalist is not "born to shop." Find the resources, create relationships with personal shoppers, and let them do the work. She can accommodate the look, budget, and time constraints, turning a chore into a pleasure.
- Specialty stores are a must. Department stores usually have entire departments for this wardrobe personality. Contemporary sporty to classic casual designers create for all the variations on this American woman theme.
- She enjoys buying local accessories and indulgences while vacationing in far off places.
- Forget discount shopping. It's a waste of time. She is not a "hit or miss" kind of gal.

The Explorer Naturalists are team players. They are loyal, faithful friends, business owners, and employees. They are dependable and responsible people. Every organization and family is blessed to have her. She is the rock, providing a firm foundation and stability for all who know her. She enjoys life to the fullest and loves to be a guest at her own party. Her guests realize this, so expectations are low and everyone joins in to create a great event. If there is a secondary personality present, it will be seen in her persona. The Explorer Naturalist blends beautifully, effortlessly with them all. In the workplace, they are hard workers, upbeat, and supportive and offer good insight, able to get to the heart of any situation.

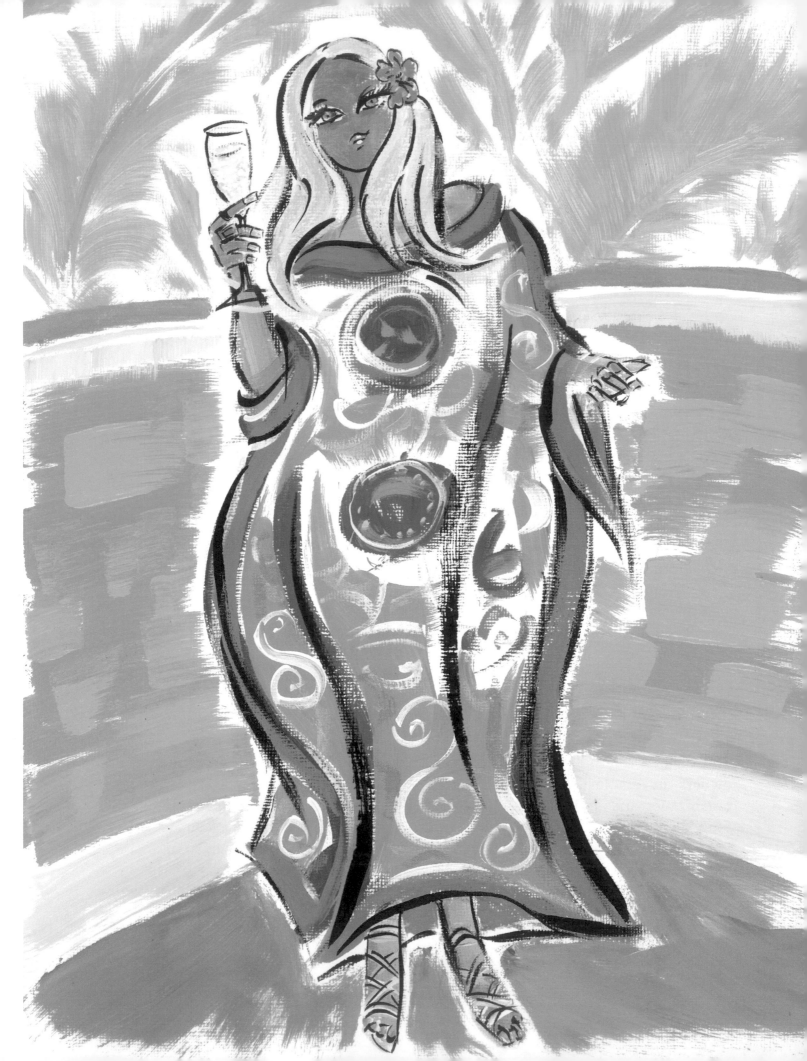

# CHAPTER 16
## The Hopeful Romantic

### The Spiritual Persona

The Hopeful Romantic's life work is to be love, do love, and spread love throughout her universe by creating moments, collecting souls, and cherishing things that beckon the dreamy bygone days and otherworldliness of femininity, heart strings, symphonic revelations, and gorgeous relationships. Her life is a never-ending series of luscious and luxe experiences. She may truly live in a dream world. She is willing to take you for the ride and bring you to neverland, where she will bathe you in belief.

She will return you to the naive notion that everything is beautiful and everyone can live happily ever after. Her mission is to create beauty and love moments for everyone she encounters, even briefly. She is a fountain of warmth and acceptance, and a lover of the romantic. She is a throwback, even in the most modern rendition, giving herself away by sharing her passion for the bucolic, pastoral, urbane, and coastal nostalgia in every imaginable fashion.

The Hopeful Romantic inspires others to stop and smell the roses along the journey, encouraging others to truly feel the glorious emotional and love language that permeates every human experience. She is an advocate and catalyst for creating connections between hearts and curating each occasion as a celebration and touchstone for adding meaning and purpose to one's life.

The Hopeful Romantic exudes charisma, femininity, and sexiness found most commonly in romantic comedies, epic films, and grand literary pieces. Her playful, flirtatious ways and sunny disposition make her irresistible to anyone within her reach. Her curves and her temperament are real. Charming, enchanting, and magnetic, she is a mistress of seduction and sensuality. She can be tremendously compassionate, sensitive, and generous in heart and spirit. She gets her feelings hurt frequently because she lives without boundaries. She loves parties and pretty things: sparkles, glitters, bows, and ephemera.

She has a keen intuition and is truly an empathetic soul, which gives her great insight into people and situations. She can be a generous hostess and employer. She flourishes wherever people and causes are in the forefront. She can also be found in the creative and culinary industries.

She is a sensualist at heart and gives great attention to all elements of taste, touch, and smell. Aesthetics and visual appeal are very important to her and provide great joy. Beautiful decor, candlelight, music, and floral scents will enhance her environment and experience.

There is an irresistible quality about her that gives the ability to influence decisions and attitudes. She is not confrontational in her approach. She prefers an indirect, softer conversation, accented with a smile and cajole. Manipulative? Yes. No one seems to mind. She can have anything her heart desires. She embraces life as it should be, a party, and believes that if you do what you love, everything else will fall into place!

## Visual Grammar

The Hopeful Romantic's fashion style is all about luxe and loveliness. Her wardrobe teems with silks, brocades, velvets, and bespoke laces. She loves exaggerated silhouettes, intricate embellishments, and vintage treasures. She paints infused romantic masterpieces with her wardrobe and wears each "art to wear" ensemble with compassion, inner joy, and kindness. She is lovely to look at and delightful to hold. The Hopeful Romantic is an altruist, vulnerable, and naive in purpose. She will not let the world's callousness affect her happiness. She chooses love again and again. If, perchance, she comes off a bit standoffish and slightly steely, it's to protect her super-soft center and aching heart.

The Hopeful Romantic glows in cinched waistlines, caftans and voluminous skirts. She often shows off her soft and voluptuous décolleté and slightly rounded and hourglass physique. She loves flow in life and fashion, refusing to appear hurried at any time. Even if she's going a million miles an hour and multitasking beyond human capacity, she always has time for tea with a friend or happy hour with her cognoscente. She is an extraordinary hostess for 1 or 100. Her doors are always open and her extensive wardrobe suits each and every occasion.

More of a dress and skirt girl, the Hopeful Romantic can wear slacks, accessorizing them in the utmost of charm and lady likeness. She wants the world to know that living slowly and relishing every moment is the key to a happy, healthy, and charmed life. She

*The Hopeful Romantic's life work is*
*to be love, do love, and spread love*
*throughout her universe*
*by creating moments,*
*collecting souls, and*
*cherishing things that beckon*
*the dreamy bygone days and*
*otherworldliness of femininity,*
*heart strings, symphonic revelations,*
*and gorgeous relationships.*

creates time capsules and invites her guest to take a ride to the sublime and softer side of life. She is an accessory lover... hats, shoes, bags, jewelry... pearls and rhinestones, diamonds and filigree. If it's vast and delicate, she is hooked!

There is a flip side to this beatific creature. Occasionally, she may let the world in to see the exotic and erotic side of her inner nature. Although it lies deeply hidden in the mermaid and siren's underwater caverns, she has a mysterious and alluring come-hither glance that exposes her fantasy world and secret garden, where she gives in to her bon vivant, exquisite, daring nature. An invitation into her secret world might shock you, making her close friends and family blush. SHHH... just blame it on the wine!

# The Earthly Being

- Height is average: 5'7" and under, occasionally taller
- Balanced, round, soft, and shapely
- Bust is full
- Defined waist, full hips and thighs

**Facial Features**
- Attractive, soft and rounded, heart shaped
- Eyes are often large and flirty or almond
- A natural feminine beauty even without makeup.

**Hairstyle**
- Length can be shoulder length, longer, or short
- Softly curled layers, feathered or blown out
- Bounce, sheen, and softness, never blunt, too straight, or stringy

# Wardrobe Style

**Key Elements**
- Think romance. She is voluptuous by night, utterly feminine and soft by day.
- Soft, flowing fabrics enhance a Romantic's beautiful curves
- Prints and florals work like a charm
- Waist-accentuating dresses are usually the best choice
- Empire waists can also be very flattering
- Iconic shirt waists, sweetheart cuts, and knits cut on the bias with flow at the hemline are great choices
- Caftans and hostess dressing

**Clothing Styles**
- Rounded lines and nonrestrictive shapes accentuate the beauty of this style persona
- Flowing with soft gathers and sometimes intricate lines with delicate ornate detailing
- Maintain fluidity from head to toe in order to elongate the silhouette, accentuate gracefulness and poise
- Waist definition is important even in suiting and jackets. The focal point of every ensemble has an anchor piece—a key piece that inspires and connects the rest of the look.
- Softness in details around the face
- Necklaces should be softly draped or curved to lay flat on the decollate
- Shoulders should not be tailored or straight. They should be rounded and curved. Tucks and gathers create softness.

**Fabrics**
- Light- to medium-weight fabrics
- Bias cut and softly draped with occasional ruching
- Finishes should be rich and luscious
- Wears silks, velvets, brocades, sweater knits, soft wools, jerseys, angoras, cashmeres, and suedes
- Chiffon and lace are fabulous for evening
- Prints include florals of varying size and design, polka dots, feather shapes, interior design elements and architectural renderings

**Accessories**
- Jewelry should be dainty to medium size in detail but lavish in effect
- Day and evening looks can be Victorian, Baroque, ornate, bordering on Rococo
- Diamonds are this girl's best friend!
- Silk flowers and scarves add a lovely touch
- Statement earrings are the final touch to garments that are heavily decorated with beautiful buttons, stitching, and embellishments such as pearls, sequins, and rhinestones
- Shoes and purses always add a touch of softness. Pliable leathers are lovely with a touch of sparkle.
- Belts should never shorten the waist (many Romantics are high-waisted). Make sure the belt width is in proper proportion.

**Unflattering Choices**
- Clothes that cheapen the appearance
- Clothes that are railroaded—cut straight on the fabric
- Symmetrical shapes and severe silhouettes
- Tailored, straight, sharp, and horizontal lines
- Rough textures

# Shopping Tips

- Consignment boutiques, resale shops, and curated collections are the best places to find treasures
- Certain ready-to-wear designers cater to this style persona. Numerous designers create collections, in extended sizes, that celebrate the Hopeful Romantic.

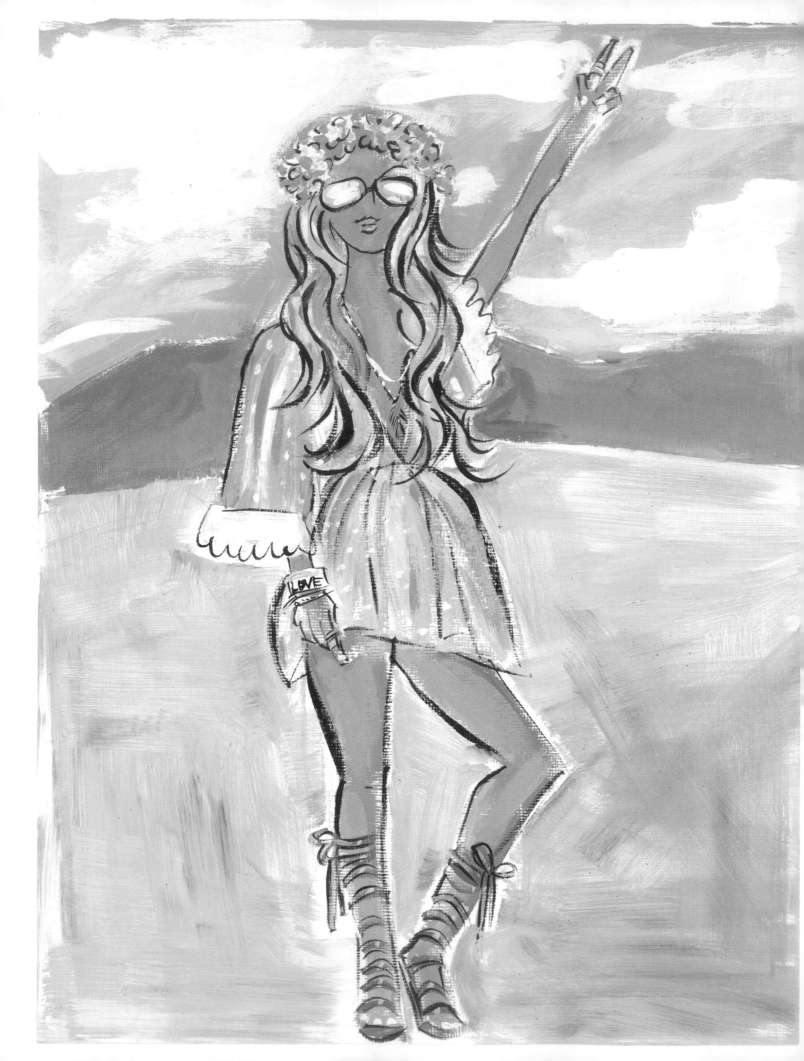

# CHAPTER 17
## The Carefree Casual

### The Spiritual Persona

The Carefree Casual is a perennial college student at heart. Her mantra is "Let there be peace on earth and let it begin with me." She is relaxed, nonchalant, and easygoing in her conversation and demeanor. She is a great listener and loves to laugh. The Carefree Casual's greatest asset is her attitude. Her vision for the world is a "love-in" where everyone gets along, lives their lives and supports each other without too much effort or concern. She can easily watch the world go by and deeply enjoy the view.

A Carefree Casual's lifestyle plays out in a singular vision for her authentic self. She hangs a "no drama" sign at her door and often sacrifices what she wants for group happiness. She is unassuming and slightly bedraggled...which becomes her most endearing quality. She uses it often to disarm hostile situations by showing up slightly late, with a latte for everyone and a lost puppy she found along the way. How can anyone argue with that?

Since the world is always sunnier on her side of the street, people love to be in her company. She is a tree hugger and animal lover. She resolves issues in a very down-to-earth way. She rescues lots of things and keeps momentos that are sentimental to her. She is a volunteer, a great friend, and a loyal girlfriend. She likes to fly under the radar. She has more than she needs. Too much of a good thing makes her self-conscious and uncomfortable.

A Carefree Casual's style allows her to move into a situation without posing any threat and diffuses even the most hypercritical unfriendly beings. She is a throwback to the '70s flower child era on Sunday and a major triathlete on Monday. Tuesday she is doing woodwork in the shop and Wednesday she is baking cookies for her BFF. Thursday she's talking her Mom off the ledge and Friday she is preparing for Saturday's race. It seems as though this free spirit has nothing to do, but under her super smile there's a lot of road racing going on!

## The Visual Grammar

Absolute comfort and no stress dressing are the hallmark of her visual language. She speaks her truth with a no-muss, no-fuss, environmentally conscious garb - cottons and knits, jeans and loose-fitting dresses. Maxi or mini, skirts and t-shirts, shorts, pants, sneakers or sandals and cool shades. She doesn't really care about her clothes lasting forever but she absolutely has her favorite pieces and will wear them until they are literally thread bare. Her lifestyle and wardrobe reflect her slightly disorganized and scattered way of being. She may be late, forget something and have the wrong address, but she shows up with a big grin and a peace offering, snacks or box wine and then the party is ready to get started. A Carefree Casual is more about lifestyle than fashion sense… she creates accidental fashion which actually look ok. She goes for hippie, cute, festival fashion, minimal or no make-up, a messy bun or long carefree hair and slightly wrinkled and appropriately mismatched garments. They could have been in her car or jammed into a drawer. Quality is not that important. Neither is fit- except when it comes to showing off her best figure assets. Bathing suits are key and special occasion wear. The rest is whatever is clean and at the top of the pile.

Her outfits allow her to move freely, speak softly and make shifts in a room or a nation without even sending up a flare. Her personality encourages change but she wants to remain anonymous. As soon as the job is finished, she often vanishes.

*The Carefree Casual*
*is a perennial college student at heart.*
*Her mantra is "Let there be peace on*
*earth and let it begin with me."*
*She is relaxed, nonchalant, and easygoing*
*in her conversation and demeanor.*
*She is a great listener and loves to laugh.*

# The Earthly Being

- 5'4" to 5'10"
- Medium to large frame
- Thin to full figure
- No bust to busty
- Spans all figure shapes
- Facial features very diverse from average oval to round to square and everything in between
- Almond-shaped eyes to round but rarely sharp
- Average lips to occasional full lips

**Hairstyle**
- Messy
- All cuts, lengths, and styles
- Mostly straight
- Occasionally "out of control" kinky curly—blame it on her genes

# Wardrobe Style

**Key Elements**
- Happy-go-lucky
- Accidental fashion sense
- Slightly wrinkled and appropriately unmatched
- She is more about lifestyle than a fashion sense...pure comfort is the key
- No muss no fuss
- Her closet and car say, "Life is like a box of chocolates. Take a bite and see what you get."
- She may throw on 20 outfits before she finally settles on the first one
- There is often a piece missing to her ensemble (lost under something or lent to a friend), which causes a bit of undue stress at showtime

**Clothing Style**
- Oversized to slightly baggy with an occasional form-fitting piece thrown in for balance
- Flannel shirts or floral "off the shoulder" peasant blouses
- Sweatshirts and pants and baby tees
- Cargo pants and a blouse or shirt or T-shirt
- Jeans and a top
- Shorts and the same tops
- Jeans, jeans, and more jeans... a pair for every occasion
- Spaghetti-strap flowy dresses, mini or maxi
- Chemises for evening if she has the figure for it

- A tailored classic casual outfit her Mom bought her for those important dates and meetings
- Coordinated work clothes—pants and a sweater or pants and a blouse
- "Athleisure" was made for her
- The same tailored outfit for interviews and Sundays
- Leggings and oversized tops

**Fabrics**
- Cotton and poly cotton blends
- Rayon, bamboo, and microfiber crepes
- Lamb's wool and nylon
- Recycled fabrications
- Earth-friendly fabrics
- Lurex and Lycra with a few sequins and occasional sparkles thrown in for good measure
- Stretchy knits

**Accessories**
- Backpack
- Earth shoes
- Sunnies
- Hats and caps
- Maybe hoop earrings or posts
- Sports watch
- Athletic shoes
- Hair ties
- Handmade bracelets
- Rings and things

## Unflattering Choices

The Carefree Casual is often passed over for opportunities, promotions, and fab potential partners who consider her an underachiever, a friend—not "date" or "relationship material." Her talents and innate qualities do not immediately shine through in first impressions. As we have learned, in our insta-society, you truly never get a second chance to make a first impression. Statistics report that the decision to swipe left or right takes less than seven seconds. This immediate critical judgment doesn't bode well for the Carefree Casual, who at first blush is a nice person but nothing to write home about!

She is underestimated, and overlooked because her wardrobe personality does not communicate confidence, ability, talent, and preparedness. She appears to lack focus and motivation and stick-to-it-ive-ness. Little do they know that under this devil-may care persona is a diamond in the rough. Yes, pretty rough. She is considered average at everything and a worker bee. What everyone seems to miss is that underneath that T-shirt a leader and a legend are waiting for their cue.

## Shopping

The Carefree Casual has great luck shopping in Junior chain stores that sell "a lot of look" for a very low price. They also find excellent mix and match items at big national brand stores and their friends' closets. Athleisure at every price is standing the test of time. This is great news for these gals who love their sweats as much as they love their dogs!

*Absolute comfort and no stress dressing are the hallmark of her visual language. She speaks her truth with a no-muss, no-fuss, environmentally conscious garb – cottons and knits, jeans and loose-fitting dresses.*

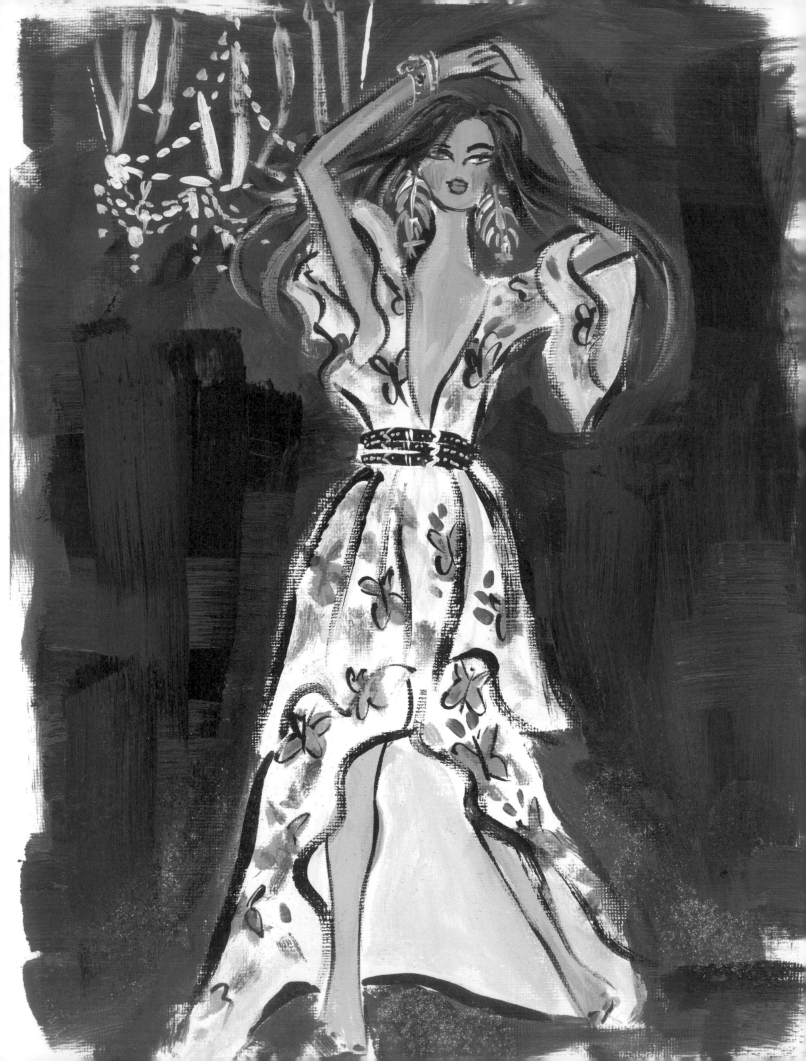

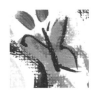

# CHAPTER 18
## *The Bohemian Rhapsody*

### The Spiritual Persona

The Bohemian Rhapsody is a highly individualistic woman whose lifestyle reflects her inner complex, seductive, astrologically charted, and highly emotional utterance. Her full immersion ode to life permeates all aspects of her daily routines. She embodies a totally unique perspective of her one precious journey, pursuing other likeminded souls to share her treasures and sip her wine. She has a passion and persuasion for fully sensory, scintillating experiences in art, music, literature, dance, design, dining, travel, philanthropy, nature, fashion, and relationships. Her life is a grand adventure or nothing at all.

Her circle of influence is mesmerized by her adventures and jumps at the invitation to participate in her gypsy glam, hippy-cum-Burning Man, Coachella-esque, flower child, earth mother, goddess, warrior, and soothsayer mystique. She is effusive and extravagant, intoxicating and fantastical. She captures her audience and transports them into her rapturous, crystal ball domain, dancing 'til dawn and fully enjoying the rapture is her mission.

### The Visual Grammar

The Bohemian Rhapsody style persona is a study in juxtaposition and jumping for joy. She is a visual clash of prints, patterns, eras, and embellishments. This Bohemian believes more is better, creating her outfit based upon her sign, celestial reading, intuitive nature, and job du jour. She spans all time and space, all eras and walks of life. She's lots of retro rolled into one collage of authentic self-expression.

The Bohemian woman is an anomaly, a throwback, a spirited and spirit-filled being. Her clothes create an experience for the observer and seem to cast a spell on her audiences. Movement is extremely important to a Bohemian. She must not be

*This Bohemian believes more is better, creating her outfit based upon her sign, celestial reading, intuitive nature, and job du jour.*

restrained in any way as she is art in motion. Her world is her palette and it is jam-packed with sights, sounds, and textures. She likes aromas and exquisite lighting... sunrises and sets, music of all types, and food from around the world. Entertainment is her passion play, as she exudes an authentic earthly sensuality and seductive nature. She puts a spell on you... and calls you mine!

From feathers and leather, skintight leggings and jeans, to volumes of gauze and gossamer, juxtaposed prints of any nature, corsets and headbands, maxi dressing to exposed skin, the Bohemian Rhapsody is ablaze in mazes of earth tones and rich jewel tones. She adores natural fabrics and piles of accessories and ephemera. You will never win playing spin the bottle with this babe. She has hundreds of layers to shed... and then all of a sudden... she's standing with a candle in her birthday suit!

Depending upon her archetype, a Bohemian Rhapsody's specific wardrobe style may range from a more conservative style persona with a singular accent to "full effect" Moulin Rouge gypsy siren. She always wears a hint of her essence, whether it be perfume, the purse, blouse, shoes, or boots. Although she conforms as she occasionally must, her authentic style language will pop out and speak to the ears that are open to hear for her song.

# The Earthly Being

- All heights, sizes, figure types
- More often, fuller figured with ample bustline
- Also see very slim women with great legs and good height

**Facial Features**
- Oval, rounded, or classic chiseled with high cheekbones
- Large, expressive eyes

**Hairstyle**
- Lots of long, straight, curly, or wavy hair
- Rich color and texture
- Often layered to increase volume and effect
- Slightly "out of control" on purpose

# Wardrobe Style

**Key Elements**
- Flowing and oversized
- Slim-fit jeans or leggings or slacks with oversized flowy blouse or kimono, jacket, sweater, or coat
- Beads and bangles, sequins, leather, feathers, and lace-excessive details
- Mixed multi-patterns from florals, paisleys, geometrics, tribal, and harem
- Over-accessorized—those earrings, though…
- Boots of all types and strappy sandals
- Movement is key to every ensemble… she wants to create a dance with her wardrobe

**Clothing**
- Jeans
- Peasant blouses
- Leggings
- Oversized tops
- Maxi dresses with asymmetrical embellished lines
- Mini dresses of similar nature if the figure allows
- Defined waist or empire waist
- Belting
- Clashes of color
- Rich autumn tones to pastel summer faded hues
- Ethnic patterns
- Stand-alone wardrobe pieces accessorized to an extreme
- All kinds of boots for every season
- Sandals with a gypsy motif

**Fabrics**
- Chiffons, georgette, crepes
- Suede and leather
- Fringe, lace, patches, embroidery, tassels
- Knits and crochet pieces
- Cottons and poly or rayon blends
- Shearling
- Faux or real fur

**Accessories**
- Bangle bracelets
- Hoop or dangle earrings
- Long chains with talismans, chokers, cameos
- Crystals, mystical icons, fetishes, beads
- Belts
- Headbands, scarves, and hats

## Unflattering Choices

- There are simply too many visual distractions, making it hard to focus on the powerful woman wearing the alluring frocks.
- Excessive layering causing unflattering angles and looking disorganized, disheveled, and unkempt.
- No figure focal point can make her appear lost in the visual circus.
- Sometimes considered to dress inappropriately for specific occasions that call for a more serious, conservative image

## Shopping Tips

There has been a strong renaissance for this look, so there are possibilities everywhere and at every price range—from couture houses to discount outlets. The malls have a strong presence for the Bohemian Rhapsody, as do festivals, flea markets, and consignment shops.

*She has a passion
and persuasion
for fully sensory,
scintillating experiences in art,
music, literature, dance,
design, dining, travel, philanthropy,
nature, fashion,
and relationships.*

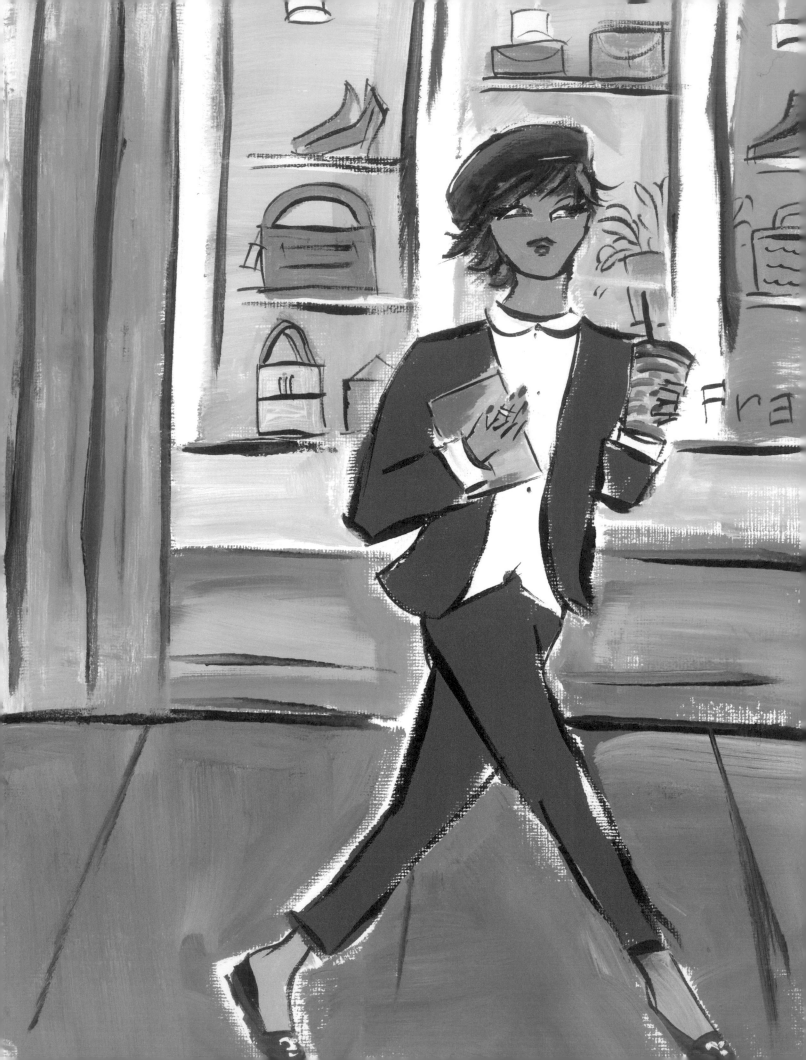

# CHAPTER 19
## The Energetic Sprite

The Energetic Sprite is characterized by her vivacious, sometimes precocious personality and is known for positivity, enthusiasm, and extraordinary energy packed into a very petite package. She is fully engaged in every conversation and at times impatient and too quick for her own good. Having said that, she is a fabulous friend, loyal and fiery, and immediately captures the room with her laughter and wit. She dazzles, sparkles, and shines wherever she goes. All this is packed into a very small frame with a very big heart!

The Energetic Sprite is a fantastic industrious worker and passionate participant in anything that interests her. Her wardrobe must contain her energy and express the scope of her being, which is truly challenging, as she is uncontainable and hard to catch! The Energetic Sprite's mission is to take action and accomplish all that she can in the time she has available.

Just looking at her pace can wear the average woman out. Her wheels are always spinning and her body is always moving, as she gets more done in a day than mere humans accomplish in a week. Highly motivated and skilled, this gal makes up in ability and capability what she lacks in height. She is fairylike, super bright, articulate, and witty. Some call it magic. I call it willpower. Many Energetic Sprites are business owners and solo entrepreneurs. Their careers span many fields and their talent and personality easily lend themselves to adapting to situations and circumstances quickly. They have answers...and are problem solvers traveling at warp speed.

This woman's worldview is quite different from the others, as she asks for forgiveness rather than permission; and with an infectious smile, sparkly eyes, and shrugged shoulders, who can resist? She has her foibles and flaws just like the rest of us... but they will be quickly disregarded because she brings so much change and motion to the party!

## Visual Grammar

Because of her petite build, and intense self-awareness, her wardrobe needs to communicate her mission and express her focus without being overpowering. Her figure ranges from angular and sharp to curvy and round. She can be proportionate but often is not even and well distributed. The Sprite wardrobe must fit her like a glove, elongate her, and highlight the features that she loves the most.

Because there is no room for error here, literally, fit and proportions are key to creating a second skin that communicates her message without upstaging her presence. Petites usually have trouble finding the perfect fit and usually have to rely upon the skills of expert tailors and alterations to fully pull off their best image. Many Energetic Sprites try to get away with wearing "off the rack," ill-fitting garments and wind up looking like they are wearing hand-me-downs. Invest in the tailoring. Trust me, it's worth it. Great-fitting clothes exude intelligence, confidence, and capability. Poorly fitting clothes convey insecurity, disorganization, untimeliness, sloppiness, and a lack of ability. Regardless of your personality type... the clothes make the woman and the fit tells the world that you are accomplished, successful, competent, and able!

The Sprite is the most misunderstood wardrobe personality. Many spend far too much time and energy trying to fit into one of the other personalities. The reason these high-octane girls are in a quandary is twofold: She possesses tremendous talent and energy. She if fun and focused. She also is jam-packed into a petite body—snappy and chic! Oftentimes, Sprites subconsciously reject their petite stature and try to become a larger persona. This always fails because if she does not accept her fab form and celebrate her unique place in fashion status, she will end up looking like little girls who are playing dress-up in their mom's closet. I suggest that The Energetic Sprite embrace the DNA and commit to create a visual grammar that fits her style, personality, and size.

The Energetic Sprite personality is not a "mini me" version of her sisters. She is a stand-alone and a standout! Her style is more classic than Bohemian; however, the fabrications change. Broken staccato patterns and lively colors convey her enthusiasm and brightness. She can be vivacious and dynamic in her wardrobe and demeanor. Spunky, energetic, enthusiastic, dazzling, and determined are adjectives that describe her persona. She's a doer with a mission and her wardrobe has to provide the visuals to convey her character.

*The Energetic Sprite is characterized by her vivacious, sometimes precocious personality and is known for positivity, enthusiasm, and extraordinary energy packed into a very petite package.*

## Earthly Being

- 5'5" or under
- Small to medium frame
- Straight, very slim, and taut, or chunky and stocky
- Curvy or angular

**Facial Features**

- If slim, they are angular
- Cheeks and chin can be round and small
- Many have a turned-up nose
- Face and eyes are animated and expressive

**Hairstyle**

- Short, cropped, boyish, or bobbed
- Can be layered with bangs
- Sassy and energetic
- Low maintenance

**Makeup**

- Less is more
- Pick a feature to focus on and keep the rest of the face much more natural and subtler
- No makeup works well on good skin except for evening—add some lip and mascara at the very least

# Wardrobe Style

**Key Elements**
- Close and accurate fit to the smallest detail
- Jacket, blouse, and skirt lengths must be in absolute proportion to overall height
- Fabrics must be fine in texture—nothing too bulky

**Clothing Style**
- Lines should be tailored and straight for a slim figure
- The silhouette must be precise, fitted for the energetic and agile
- Patterns and colors should be animated and smaller
- Snappy, chic designs with lots of contrasted trims, braided trims, or beading. Military styles work well.
- Contemporary designs work best to avoid the dowdy look
- Details and accessories should be small, sharp, eye-catching, but not overpowering
- Styles must be energetic and compact in proportion and line
- Fit must be perfect
- A pure Sprite reflects the Eternal Beauty style in shapes and lines but not in color, fabrication, and pattern
- An angular, straight, thin Sprite can wear more dramatic looks and shapes as long as the scale is adjusted to her height
- A softer, rounder, bustier Sprite can be more romantic in her selections. Again, fit is key.
- Her clothes must convey decisiveness, candor, intelligence, speed, and joie de vivre, mirroring her persona
- The hemline must be at the knee or slightly above—elongates the leg. Long skirts are disastrous at best.
- Jacket lengths must be short, waist jackets, or slightly over the hipbone—never longer or legs will look too short and torso too long

**Fabrics**
- Colors are bold and sassy
- Multicolor splashes and caricatures work fine
- Prints should be contemporary and can be geometric and abstract
- Fabric must be crisp and hold its shape
- Surfaces are smooth and refined
- Matte and low-luster textiles work best
- Weights are light- to medium-oriental silks, damasks, crisp cottons, twills, or wool gabardines. Synthetic blends are great too!
- Evening fabrics should be sleek with tailored features and angular necklines. Even asymmetrical hemlines will be great. Crisp metallics and beading also suit this figure well.

*She is fairylike, super bright,*
*articulate, and witty.*
*Some call it magic. I call it willpower.*

**Accessories**
- Jewelry must be to scale: nothing big and chunky
- Jewelry should be crisp, geometric, asymmetrical, or irregular—even colorful
- Contrasting hosiery and leggings are fabulous
- Dark hose must be sheer

## Unflattering Choices

- Monochromatic color schemes that sap energy
- Neutrals
- Florals and drapes
- Oversized and unstructured garments
- Rough textures
- Sheer, delicate fabrics
- Frills and blousons
- Antique, artisan, and intricate designs

## Shopping Tips

- The petite department is her shopping destination
- Mix and match dressing is great but with a slightly more classic finish
- Coordinate two or three colors in an outfit—a dominant, a neutral, and an accent
- Capsule dressing is a great strategy
- Accessorize with the dominant color
- Shoes must not be too clunky or overpowering, throwing look off balance
- Boots are not great because they make the legs appear shorter

The Energetic Sprite will be perennially young at heart. Many Energetic Sprites are still taking the world by storm into their 80s and above. Carpe diem! A young Sprite might not be taken seriously since she looks younger than her age for a long time. My advice is to go with it. Better to look young and surprise them than to try to look older and simply look ridiculous.

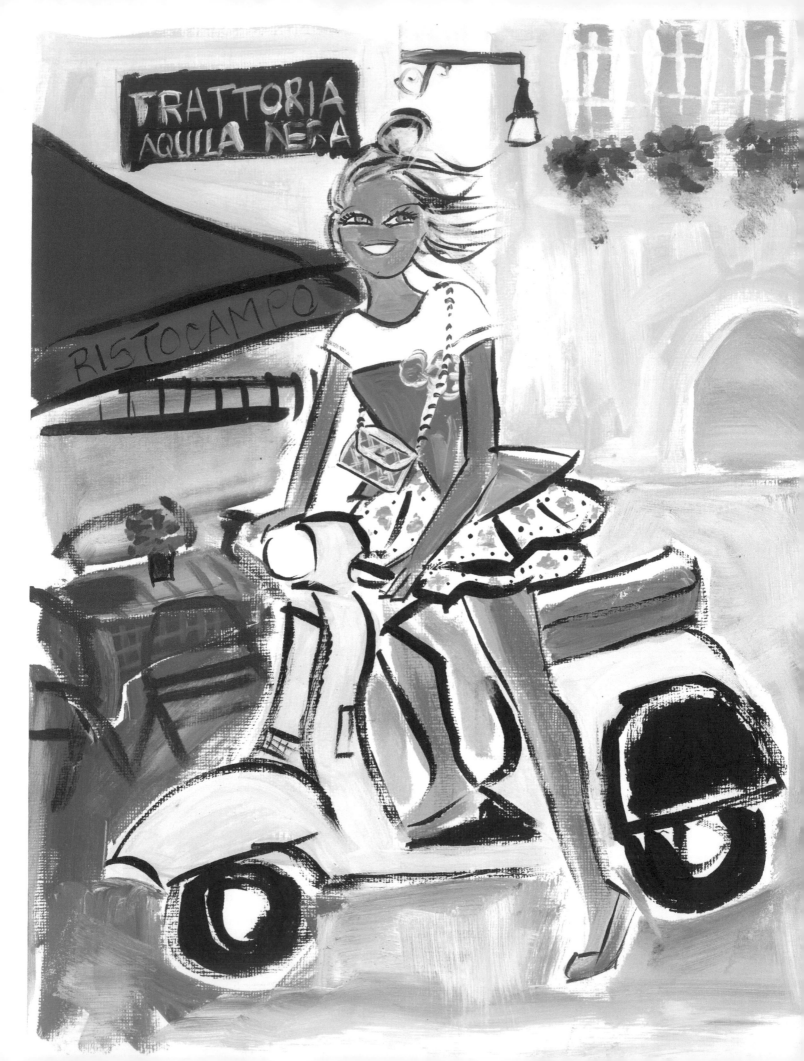

# CHAPTER 20
## The Ingenue Muse

### The Spiritual Persona

The Ingenue Muse used to be the girl who dated the class president, married the prince, and had a secret garden. Today she may be heading up her own finance company or the CEO of her own not-for-profit... she may be starring in the school play or the sweetheart of Sigma Chi. The Ingenue Muse may become the eternal beauty as she ages or she may remain an ageless ingenue forever. It's more about her spontaneous and contagious joy, small frame, and mischievous magical sensibilities.

The Ingenue Muse is a bit of a rebel with a lot of decorum, obligatorily carrying out the family name and traditions while imprinting onto society the crest and graciousness of her clan. She is the belle of the ball and balances a heavy weight of lineage in her heart as if they were books upon her head. She, like her grown-up counterpart, the Eternal Beauty, was born to exemplify immaculate style, polish. and panache. Her wardrobe style is simple and well-tailored, delicate fabrications as to not weigh her spirit down, along with neat lines and silhouettes to best frame her pretty face and sweet demeanor.

Her figure is slight and easily overwhelmed, so solid colors with a focused pattern in small scale work best. She can dress like a princess with hoops and yards of tulle and duchesse satin or she can pull off Audrey's ballet flats, Capri pants, and white shirt. She is a beautiful budding rose who refuses to be clipped and placed in a crystal vase.

### Visual Grammar

Simplicity and sophisticated classic styling look best on the Ingenue. She is the muse of designers who embrace youth and status. Her carriage is perfect. Her waist is small. Her hips are slight and her neck is elongated. Doleful eyes and a porcelain complexion complete the vision. You can spot her from a mile away.

The Ingenue Muse personality is embodied within the debutante avatar. She is light and whimsical, impetuous and shy. She may be a contradiction of terms, but one thing is sure, she is sweet and girlish, pretty, poised, and mannerly.

The Ingenue Muse shares her sister's romantic nature but not her physique. She is a youthful, innocent portrait of femininity. She is not overtly sexy. She is demure and non-threatening and is often thought to need protection from the world. The Ingenue is often not taken too seriously. Beware! Underneath that gentle persona lies a bright, articulate, passionate, and stubborn spirit who is led by curiosity, conviction, and duty. She keeps her thoughts to herself most of the time and lives in a beautiful fantasy world where princes ride in on horses to save the day and sweep her away to happily ever after. She is like a beautiful butterfly in flight. Her demeanor and naïveté are communicated in her wardrobe choices.

The Ingenue Muse is a bit puzzling – spirited but sensible, adorable yet erudite, slapstick funny, and quietly demure, the center of attention and the girl who hides behind her laptop with a pencil in her hair. She is very bright, knows silence is golden, but can be a bit fiery and outspoken when necessary. Her dance card is full and so is her imagination and secret longing to explore everything and everywhere. Her clothing style reflects her paradox. There is an outfit for every occasion and a persona to go with it. She surprises the world with her fluency in all things fashion and conversation. She is a fairy… just don't try to clip her rapidly fluttering wings.

## Earthly Being

- Height is 5'7" and under
- Feminine, small boned, soft, straight, dainty
- Delicate stature, regardless of height
- Figure slightly boyish, small busted, flat stomach and derriere

**Facial Features**
- Cheeks rounded, chin rounded, or tapered
- Eyes are large and innocent
- Fine boned
- Delicate coloring

**Hairstyle**
- Longer hair can be pulled back or slightly curled
- Shorter hair can be feathered, or even pixie cut
- Updos, French twists, and knots

*The Ingenue Muse personality is embodied within the debutante avatar. She is light and whimsical, impetuous and shy. She may be a contradiction of terms, but one thing is sure, she is sweet and girlish, pretty, poised, and mannerly.*

## Wardrobe Style

**Key Elements**
- All things Audrey
- Retro '50s sorority style or rebel
- The "boyfriend" look works for ultra-casual
- '60s mod
- Small prints
- Defined waistlines and cropped pants
- Lots of detailing
- Feminine and refined
- Retro debutante

**Clothing Style**
- Frills, ruffles, lace, and delicate finishes suit her best
- Small, delicate florals and prints that do not overwhelm her diminutive frame
- Embellishments are perfect as long as they are not overpowering
- Sweetheart necklines, Peter Pan colors, fitted sweaters, and boat necks are all flattering
- Pencil skirts to full circle skirts and tulle
- Close-fitting, straight-legged trousers, leggings, or capris
- Sweater sets and ballet flats
- Kitten heels and librarian glasses
- Sweetly elegant and classic for evening... not too serious and not too sexy

**Fabrics**
- Lightweight soft woolens, angora, cashmere, fine silk, crisp cotton, batistes, voile, crochet, jersey, fine knits, piques, light satins, microfibers, twill, or duck

**Accessories**
- Jewelry is soft and dainty—nothing overpowering
- Feminine florals, ribbons, bows, cameos, pearls, and lingerie
- Neat shoes, ballet flats, pumps, open-toes, stilettos, strappy sandals, and canvas sneakers

## Unflattering Choices

- Large patterns and disproportionate prints
- Over-the-top design will overpower The Ingenue Muse
- The older Ingenue must avoid dressing too young even though she can still fit into junior clothes. She can rapidly become a fashion disaster.

*The Ingenue Muse*
*is a bit puzzling—*
*spirited but sensible,*
*adorable yet erudite,*
*slapstick funny,*
*and quietly demure,*
*the center of attention*
*and the girl who hides*
*behind her laptop*
*with a pencil in her hair.*

# Shopping Tips

- A little goes a long way! Keep in mind that the Ingenue figure can be easily overpowered. Fit must be impeccable. Line has to be soft to soft straight but not rigid. Fabrication has to be soft to moderate. Pattern has to be small, if at all.
- Do the homework and find designers who tailor clothes to the Ingenue figure and style consciousness. Because the body frame is small, fit can be tough, especially if the woman is taller than average. Contemporary departments and Juniors will sometimes work best.
- Spring and summer are her favorite shopping seasons.
- Fabric quality is not crucial although a few key luxe pieces are always advisable. Most wardrobe pieces can be "a lot of look." An Ingenue can afford an expensive wardrobe if each price point is kept in the moderate range. There are so many fashion personas she can wear and enjoy! The professional wardrobe should be more investment dressing and the accessories that go with it should be classic. Have fun! Be charming! Borrow from the Eternal Romantic sister—the fashion world is her oyster! Dive in!

An Ingenue Muse might say, "I don't care what you think of me... I don't think of you at all." Her vulnerability allows her to move between the world stages with an incredible lightness of being. However, she is often gossiped about and ostracized because she is simply too good to be true! To counter these false claims and attacks on her purity and altruistic sensibilities, she sometimes takes chances that lead down a path out of the secret garden and into the wild world! She seems to get through it all but she certainly gets her shares of "Bless your heart."

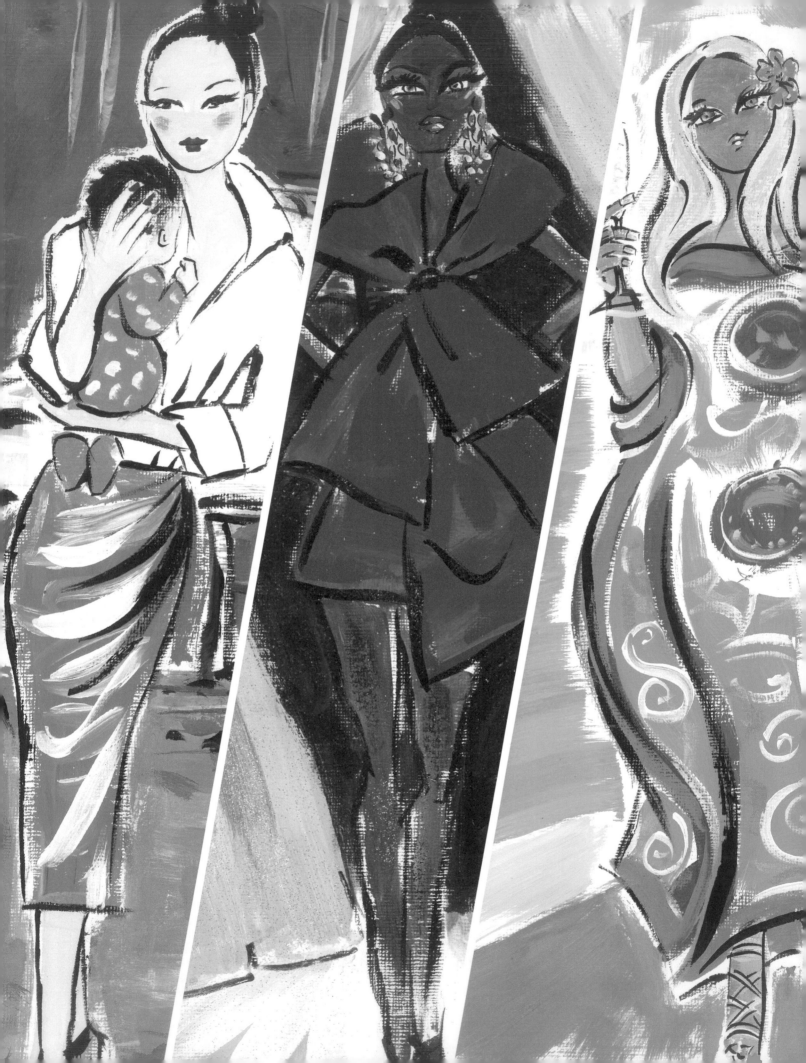

# CHAPTER 21
## *The Combination Style Personas and Summary*

### The Hybrid Style Personas

Although many women fall into a singular persona, there are some who truly have Combination Style Personas. Whether it's by nature or by choice, these women alternate between two or more styles, often wearing one style for day and another for evening. Other times, hybrid personalities emerge when the dominant type is determined by the physical attributes (structure/body type/hair/facial features and style preferences) while the secondary personality is determined by those features that are not in alignment with the dominant type and not aligned with your personality traits. Today fashion is a veritable coat of many colors, lengths, styles, fits and fabrics. There is something for every mood and persona – have fun with it!

Hopefully, after reading this book, you will truly discover and embrace your fashion formula and create wardrobes that will leave the world in awe of your presence. Your checkbook will be astounded by your intelligence and your heart fully confident that there is something at your fingertips to wear for who you want to be today. These combination style personas are for everyone. Some women fully articulate their beings in the variations of one style voice. Other personalities truly embody their inner nature best by having other voices create a gorgeous harmonic chord in each solo performance.

For example, the Eternal Beauty is classic in her personal style preferences and falls into the physical attributes that help determine her classification. There can be hybrid personas that emerge from time to time in her character that enable her to expand her clothing options to include flavors from the other personalities to suit her mood or means for the day. Let's say that she is flying to a fabulous ski resort for a week of skiing, après ski, and spa. She might decide to augment her style by adding some Explorer Naturalist pieces to her wardrobe so that she looks and feel fabulous wherever she roams in her winter wonderland.

Or let's say that elegant gal has decided to step up her visual image for her new corporate or charitable board position and needs to create a more commanding and powerful persona. She would do well to add a bit of Entrance Maker into her classic look, whether it be in color or silhouette, to bring forward her more dominant nature.

To clarify, some women will truly have two style personas and are really a blend of each. All of us can adopt elements from each person and add them to our wardrobe to expand our visual horizons and take a little stroll on the style wild side! Nothing better than to keep your admirers guessing, girls!

The key to exploring these other style personas successfully is never compromise fit for fashion. If your clothes don't fit perfectly, the image they portray will undermine all else. Wearing clothes that are ill fitting gives the impression that one might be disorganized, sloppy, possessing a low self-esteem, untimely, and incapable. Well-fitting clothes convey intellect, confidence, capability, attention to detail, and respect for self and others. Fit is queen. So is line and proportion. Fit must be your first consideration all the time, for you know what they say about the shoe...

No matter how many elements you add to your wardrobe possibilities, never stray too far from your style persona truth... That old adage still rings true, ladies.... I can still hear my Mother saying, "You never get a second chance to make a first impression." I will only add... make it your best!

*There can be hybrid personas that emerge from time to time in her character that enable her to expand her clothing options to include flavors from the other personalities to suit her mood or means for the day.*

## Summary

The most important factor to consider before you leave your home and take that peek in the mirror and check your teeth is, "Am I authentic? Do I look like who I am? Is my outfit sending out a clear and confident image? Does it nonverbally convey my strengths and does it assist me in the tasks that I am facing today? Will my wardrobe assist me in succeeding? Am I dressed appropriately for the occasion? Do I look good from all angles? How about my shoes and accessories? How about my bag? How is my hair and makeup?

If you can honestly give yourself high marks in every area, you must deeply feel that you have the whole world wrapped in your arms today and are empowered, and positive that you will experience joy, success, and abundance. Your wardrobe informs your image. Your image reflects your personal brand. Your presence speaks volumes before you say a word.

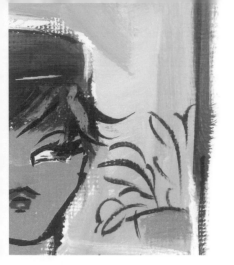
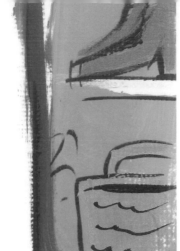
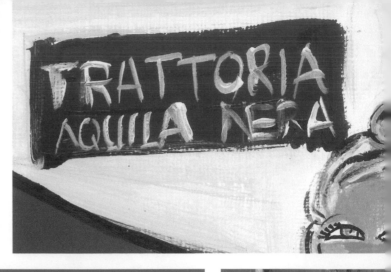

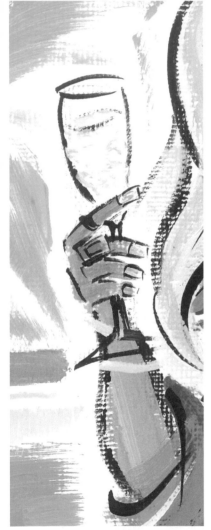

> *Choose fewer and choose well – in Champagne, in life, and in clothing.*

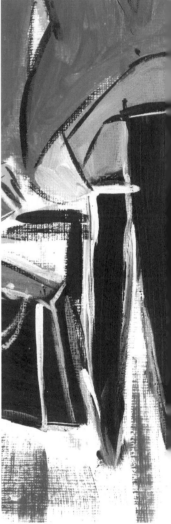

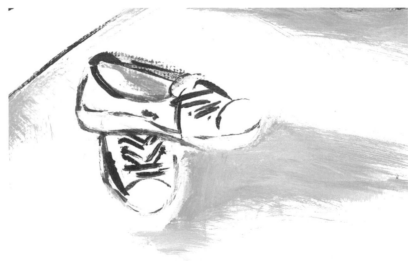

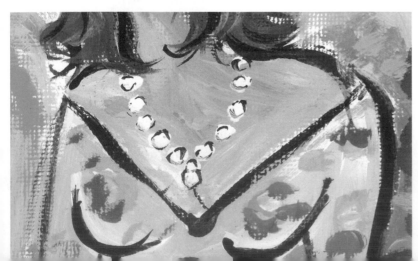
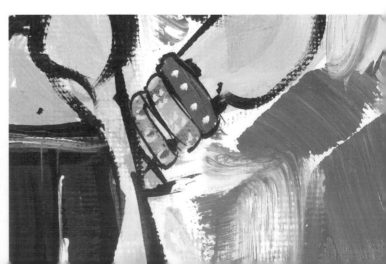

# CHAPTER 22
## It's Sort of Like Champagne

When I think about sharing the concept of quality—and how important it is in purchasing a new wardrobe—it's like talking about Champagne...another of my great passions. You can drink better or lesser brands—they both have bubbles and will get you effervescent—but one is tasting the stars and the other seeing stars when you wake up the next day with the hangover from Hades. That's the difference between quality and quantity, between dancing with the divine and saving the last dance for the guy with two left feet. Choose the one who will respect you in the morning, dears, and not leave your precious self-embarrassed and bruised. Choose fewer and choose well—in Champagne, in life, and in clothing.

Now, plenty of girls say, "I can't afford expensive Champagne or couturier. So, I drink and dress for my budget." I say, you can't afford not to drink or dress for the best. Would you rather have 25 ill-fitting dresses that you bought on sale at a cheap store that you kind of like and will fall apart in one wash? Or would you rather invest in five dresses that fit you like a glove, make you feel like a queen, last for years, and convey your authentic self to the world as an ambassador? Hmmm... okay, it's like this: Cheap wine is cheap. If you don't know the difference, it's time to step it up. If you don't care, stop drinking it. Not only does it make you look bad, it makes you feel bad about yourself. The same thing happens when you wear cheap clothes. Others will judge you and you will judge yourself.

*Enough said. A Votre Santé!*

*It's not only how others see you.*
*It's how you see yourself.*
*If you don't know better, you can't do*
*better. I will teach you to know better.*
*You must then choose to do better.*

### A String of PEARLS and a Penny for Your Thoughts

As we approach the finale and afterparty of your journey to dressing for your highest and best self, there are several pearls of wisdom— 20 exactly—that I would like to offer you, glorious girl! It's sort of like my gift with purchase to you.

It's all about shopping. I think that I was born in a department store... *nearly*.... Yes, my family is six generations deep in discriminating and discerning shopping and styling across the globe. My budget doesn't always match my taste but my style will never suffer, and neither should yours. Now that you are equipped with all the tools and knowledge necessary to shop like a pro and style like you were born for the runway of your life...

Here are my steadfast rules for managing the mall and your money and bubbling up in a boutique without bubbling over:

**Just Another Manic Monday:** The Best Day and time of the week to shop is Monday morning. The weekend traffic is over and the store has been refreshed! If you can't shop on Monday, then please shop in the morning before everyone is frazzled and in a frenzy.

**Combat Gear:** Look great when you shop! Wear makeup and do your hair...the clothes will look better on you and you will get better treatment. Do wear easy-to-take-off, comfortable clothes so that you do not exhaust yourself before you even start your fittings.

**Lingerie, Please!** How much lingerie do you own that is meant to be taken off? More than we can politely discuss today. And how many real panties and bras do you have in your drawer? That's what I thought. Oh, the fortune we spend on fantasy only to come up short when what we see in the mirror is more of a reality show than a romantic comedy. Please start shopping in the foundation department and work outwards to the clothes.

If your undies aren't supporting your mission statement, nothing is going to look good! Invest and wear a good support bra and seamless panties, and if you don't have any shapewear and need it, please buy it before you try on those body con dresses. Haven't you noticed that everything is sort of body con these days? Even a caftan requires underpinnings. And it's not a matter of size; there are lots of skinny girls who would benefit from shapewear. As time goes on, it becomes all about the innies and outies when it comes to looking tucked in and fab! A good bra will take ten years and twenty pounds off your figure... and magically your waist may appear just where you left it!

**Fit to Be Tied:** It's sort of like not settling for the table by their kitchen in a restaurant; the more room you have, the less claustrophobic you'll feel. Ask for the biggest fitting room and insist on a rear view. If the store doesn't have a three-way mirror, use your phone to see yourself from all angles. The camera doesn't lie. Lighting is usually very poor in many fitting rooms. Make sure you get out of the fitting room and into a well-lit area to reflect upon your wardrobe choice. A picture is worth a thousand words. Take it or ask the sales associate to take it for you.

**Leave Them Hanging:** I never buy anything right away. Select what you like and have the salesperson put items on hold. Leave the store, have lunch, check out the competition, and then return in your power to make the right purchasing decisions. DO NOT SUCCUMB TO PRESSURE! It's their mission to sell clothes...it is not your job to provide them with job security! Buy what's best. Leave the rest.

**Love 'Em or Leave 'Em:** Only buy what you absolutely love, what look fabulous on you! How many good deals do you have hanging in your closet with the tags still on them? Make a list. Do not get distracted. Buy what you need. Enough said.

**Quality, Not Quantity:** My formula for success is to buy less and invest in timeless, high-quality pieces and then add a few trendy pieces to update your look seasonally. Cheap clothing makes you look cheap and trust me, cheap is dear. Never settle for anything or anyone that lessens who you are in image, status, or feelings. If you look inferior, you will feel inferior. If you feel inferior, you will certainly be treated inferiorly. It's the law of the universe.

I am not going to fight with a higher power... dress in the best that you can afford. When you know better and can afford better, dress better. My grandmother taught me so many huge lessons when I was very young. She was an extraordinary fashion designer, way ahead of her time in every way! One day she said to me, "It's far better to shop at a more expensive store and buy the least expensive clothes that they carry than to buy the most expensive garment at a cheap store." OMGOSH! She is right... the quality at the better store will always be superior to the quality at the less expensive store.

**Press for Service:** Set the record straight. Ask for assistance and let them know that you are looking for these specific items, nothing more and nothing less. Alert them to your budget and preferences. The more informed your salesperson is, the less hassle the whole experience is for everyone.

**VIP:** In-store personal shopping services and stylists can become a girl's best friend! I have had longer relationships with salespeople than I have had with men.... They laugh with you, cry with you, and put your needs and wants first. On occasion, they even have bubbles and bites waiting.

Years ago, I was pressed into service to do a stint at a major luxury brand store in the dual role of Fashion and Private Shopping Club Director. I can only say that for many women, this place not only provides the highest service and kindness, it provides a safe place to bare one's soul along with the rest! When a daughter gets married, we were the first to know. When a spouse died, we closed the club to receive them. When a girl found herself back on the circuit, we were there for a total makeover and toast. When there was a major climb up the corporate ladder, we were there to create her new look to fit her new station. It is truly an awe-inspiring responsibility. I simply love to work with other stylists. There are tons of perks...sale pre-shopping, exclusivity, special promotions, special events...let's just say they make you feel special! And isn't that special?!? One word of caution...they must sell. You have a "spend" and they do intend to make sure you spend it with them.

**Stand In:** Try your outfits on with shoes.... It changes the entire line and fit of the garment. If you didn't bring shoes, ask to use a pair. They will be gladly provided.

**First Come, First Served:** Shop Presale so that you get first dibs on all the goodies you didn't or couldn't purchase at full price. One of my favorite shopping strategies is, "Buy some now, add more later." Know the lines and colors that fit you best and invest in the basic pieces in a neutral color. I usually suggest six pieces: dress, jacket, pants, blouse, skirt, and chemise. Purchase these well-fitting pieces in your size at full price. Alert the salesperson that once the rest of the collection goes on sale, you would like to complete the look with accent pieces and/or adding a complementary color. This strategy works well with designers who ascribe to capsule concept dressing..

**Get the Coupon:** Ask when a promotion is about to start. If you go online before you shop at specific stores, often they will offer you a discount on your initial purchase. Get the coupon or code and ask if it can be honored at the store. The sales staff will gladly give you a promotion start date if they know it. If you happen to get stuck paying full price for something that goes on sale within two weeks of your purchase, get a price adjustment... everyone does it.

**EAT! For Goodness Sake:** The day you decide to shop is not the day to start a crash diet. That plate has been served.... Shopping burns calories and requires stamina. Starving yourself will only result in a sugar crash, headache, and binging later. Take time to have a decent breakfast and plan on lunch or pack a snack. Many stores offer water... hydrate. It's good for the skin and for the soul. Fluids help keep you grounded.

**Only Buy Clothes That Fit You Now!** If I have heard it once I have heard it a thousand times: It fits a little snug, but after I lose 10 pounds it'll be perfect! Umm, probably not! Why set yourself up for failure and self-loathing? Buy what fits now. And if it doesn't fit, chances are it never will.

My other pet peeve is women who refuse to buy any new clothes because they are waiting until they lose weight. Really? In the meantime, is it really in your best interest? NO, IT'S NOT! As we have discovered, your self-esteem and overall success is all wrapped up in body image. It is soooo important that you dress for who you are now. Tomorrow is another day... another size. What's most important is that you honor the skin you're in today. Punishing yourself for not being at your desired weight is not supporting your cause. Be kind to yourself. Buy a few good-looking pieces for now; as you lose, buy a few more pieces. As you see your reduced self in nice-fitting and good-looking clothes, your self-esteem and confidence will skyrocket and act as a further incentive to stay on task. Celebrate each victory along the way—you are so worth it!

**Buy Complete Looks:** If you can't find the right blouse to go with the skirt at purchase, chances are you will never find it! There is still stuff in my closet that I talked myself into believing that I would find the perfect top to match! NOT! Also, if a garment isn't comfortable in the dressing room, you will never wear it. When buying pants, make sure you sit down in them. If there's one thing I cannot stand it's having pants that are cut too short in the ride! UGH! Sit, bend, and move. Make sure that the slacks, jacket, and/or dress allow you to move effortlessly.... We don't need any wardrobe malfunctions on your runway.

**If the Shoe Fits, Swear by it!** The best time to buy shoes is later in the day when your feet are the largest. Only buy what fits you well. And if you happen to have a hard-to-fit size, especially narrow, ask to try on a pair that has never been tried on before. Fat feet stretch out shoes... look for a brand-new pair. Also, when you discover a shoe that works, consider purchasing it in several colors. Shoe designers are notorious for stopping production on a particular shoe. Buy the staple in two colors. it's another chapter of investment shopping. If you can't stand for something, you will fall for anything. Two are better than one.

**Edit Your Closet Ruthlessly:** Before you go shopping, clean out your drawers and closets. If you haven't worn a piece in two years, donate it! Or resell it. Clutter causes brain fog... and none of us need to go there.

**Make Up Your Life:** Have your makeup done by a pro at least once a year to keep your look fresh and updated. Ruts are for the road, not for your face. Stay current. Ask for samples before you buy skin care... better to try it before you buy it. Also, keep the original packaging and receipt for your purchase. If you have an allergy, many stores will require the return to be in the packaging and with a receipt.

**Accessorize!** Invest in a quality bag, shoes, and a few good pieces of jewelry. Accessories can save the day, especially when traveling for work or play with a carry-on suitcase. A dress can fade, but a good pair of shoes, bag, scarf, or watch can last for decades.

I am fine with being accused of eating a tart... but never settle for being accused of being a tart. Do not shop in departments that no longer serve you. Dearests, just because some of you can fit into clothes in the Junior Department doesn't mean you should be wearing them. The curtain may have fallen on those days. Congrats on maintaining your figure but deal with the fact that it may be time to wear your big girl pants now! Age appropriateness is real. Embrace it.

**Don't Get Stuck Holding the Bag:** Check the return policy before you get stuck holding the bag. I always ask for the return policy before I buy.... If the policy doesn't suit you, maybe it's time to wear a dress. (:

*"...your self-esteem and overall success is all wrapped up in body image. It is soooo important that you dress for who you are now. Tomorrow is another day... another size."*

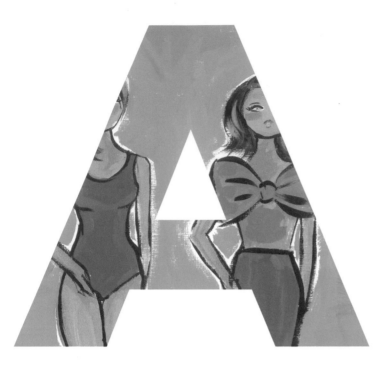
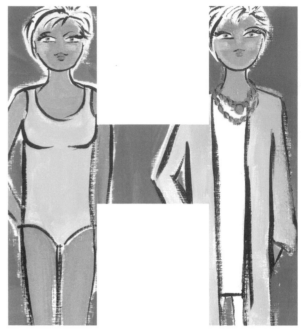
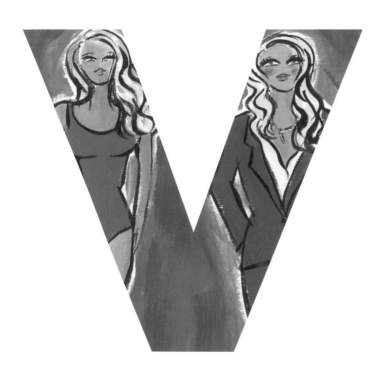
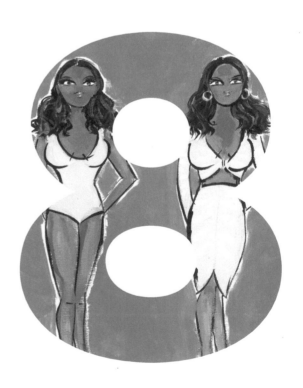

# CHAPTER 23
## A Frame by Any Other Name

Fashion is a language that speaks without concerns. It is a platform for expression and substance. Trivial and profound, it exists as singular tiles that we fashion into a gorgeous mosaic of our personal style. The pieces are quite simple: dresses, pants, chemise, foundations, accessories, and shoes. From those simple concepts we add function, fabrication and line, drape, form, and finesse. We embellish and restrain, expand, reduce, focus and distract the viewer's eye. The experience of wearing fashion should be as exhilarating and enticing as the experience of viewing fashion. A garment should feel as good as it looks on you. There is the rub. Your personal experience with fashion must be a love affair, not a detente.

Fashion has its limitations. We have expectations. It's best to explain the parameters of what we can and cannot expect from dressing for success.

The more you understand the science of what fashion can achieve and work within your personal body type, coloring, personality, and preferences, the more control you have over the outcome. The more you understand the private demands you place upon yourself in a public arena, the better able you are to incorporate self-understanding and lifestyle into the unique fashion identity you create as fashion grammar, your style DNA.

Let's begin with what clothing cannot achieve. If you are petite, clothing cannot make you tall. Knowing how to use color blocking and vertical lines can make you appear taller, but nothing can change the frame. Work with it, not against it, and witness fabulous results. Over the past many decades, it has been an honor and privilege to work with women of all ages, sizes, shapes, and situations. It has been the gift of a lifetime to watch the metamorphosis that takes place in a tiny dressing room with questionable lighting and a fixed budget.

One day, I was in the dressing room with a woman who admittedly announced that she

# Fashion has its limitations.
# We have expectations.

was a size 20. Upon our meeting, it was obvious that she underestimated her size by a few numbers. She looked at me nervously, admitting that perhaps she hadn't been totally honest in our phone conversations. She tearfully explained that she had put herself on a crash diet before flying to meet me, which backfired! She had shame and fear in her eyes, anticipating what might be another disastrous shopping encounter. She asked, "What are we going to do now?" As we stood on the corner of 5th Avenue and 40th Street on a bone-chilling, rainy NYC morning, I quickly responded, "Well, I can tell you what we are not going to do." She gasped. "We are NOT going to make you look thin!" She almost fainted...her eyes opened as wide as her mouth. Then I added, "We ARE going to make you look fabulous, but we are not going to make you look thin. Fashion cannot do that!" I gave her a huge smile and a nod of absolute assurance. She started laughing so hard she cried, and with a huge sigh of acknowledgement and relief, the pressure was off... and we set off to a day like none other. I whisked her into a cab and off we went down the rabbit hole of extraordinary adventure and amazement. After four hours, she stood in the center of the department store, gazing at herself in a full-length mirror, and started to cry again. She said, "I have never felt beautiful before in my life. Today I feel beautiful. I look beautiful and I see myself as my true nature. Thank you for giving me the most extraordinary gift... the gift of accepting my own presence with confidence and joy. Thank you so much for opening my eyes and heart to loving myself. I finally see on the outside how I feel on the inside."

Yes, a box of tissues and 22 perfectly appointed outfits later, we zoomed across town to a great salon, where we did a total hair transformation followed by makeup and brows. I taught her how to work with her very curvy body, the best part of her leg, lovely décolleté, beautiful big brown eyes, and a healthy, thick mane of hair. She was astonished. She will never be the same... and neither will her life, her relationships, and her career.

This process is miraculous and the benefits are long lasting. Let's say "Yes" to the dress that looks the best on you and forget the rest along with the script that goes with it! When you love the skin you're in, it will love you right back.

Spending a substantial amount of time in a naturist camp does wonders for a girl. We not only see how we are but we see how others are without filters or beauty apps. It's just humans living their lives in their birthday suits. I queried several Millennials who grew up vacationing there every summer with their families, whether they feel that this experience helped them develop a more positive and empowered self-image. None of them had even thought about it, but 100 percent agreed that growing up seeing people's bodies and understanding that no one is perfect and everyone has beauty and value helped to create a higher level of self-acceptance and esteem. When everyone is naked, there is no judgment based upon appearance. Without adding a second skin, a person's first skin conveys simply that although we are different, we are totally the same. We are perfect souls enjoying a totally human experience. When all that is unseen becomes seen, the thoughts and conversation become about life and love, stories and shared experiences. The pressure of looking like yourself in clothes is relieved entirely.

Once everyone is rendered naked, there seems to be a great ease and grace about the way one comports their everyday life. The trappings fade away with the sunrise and the essence of a person becomes known. Living naked is truly a paradox. There is no judgment in the raw form. Judgment begins the minute we get dressed and put on our masks, pretentions and affectations. Our wardrobe becomes our armor...and in the war of cultural ego, we prepare to win.

Coming to peace with your body type is the steppingstone for achieving serenity with the shape you cannot change and realizing that you can change the "appearance" of your shape with an eye on style and know that we are all imperfect bodies... and accepting that with your newly found understanding, your highest and best persona will emerge loud and proud!

A frame is just an adornment to the main attraction. Your body is the frame and physical manifestation of your being on earth, capturing your essence and containing it in a specific form. Let's face it, we inherited our shapes from our family. It's all in the DNA. As hard as we try to alter how we were born and the temple we are given at birth, our bodies represent who we are in the physical world. Our body shape stays with us for life. Unless of course we choose to alter it surgically to seek the balance or imbalance we perceive to be "beautiful." As they say, it is in the eye of the beholder. Discovering, understanding, and embracing your physical presence, your body and all its splendor, is the key to achieving happiness and success in creating your authentic self in your second skin, your wardrobe. The success of your relationship with your second skin has a lot to do with understanding the reality of your first skin.

Have you ever noticed that some designers just seem to "get" you not only in style but in shape? Every designer makes clothes for a specific body type. Their lines and proportions are mathematically figured into the formula for their collections, and their fit models are hired as a representative of the body frame that they seek to wear their line. Some designers have more than one line and dedicate each line to a particular physical silhouette.

Many women look into the mirror in absolute horror and loathe what they see. After forty years of witnessing the bare truth about bodies, I can say that none of us are totally satisfied with how we look. Instead of celebrating what's right about our figures, we immediately zone in on the flaws and magnify them to the max—instead of learning how to deal with our bodies like the models we see on the catwalk.
Yes, even supermodels have areas of their bodies that they would rather not discuss.

Each of us has a feature we inherited, or six, that make us feel less than a "Perfect 10." NEWS FLASH: NONE OF US ARE A PERFECT 10! We have simply mastered the art of disguise. As I have mentioned before, this is the art of bringing the viewer's eye to focus upon the features we love about our bodies and distracting them from the parts we do not love.

Developing a style is learning to wardrobe the body we were born with in such a way that we maximize its appeal with color, angles, proportions, detailing, and design. We achieve this by employing all these elements in ways that enhance our beauty and diminish our flaws. The eye, ear, mind, body, and spirit strive to achieve balance. In fashion, we use optical illusions to achieve "visual balance." This is the first secret to creating your wardrobe as art!

Now that you have identified your authentic archetype and your style persona, let's discover your genetic body type. Body types often align with a personality. Sometimes we are a blend of more than one type, in which case we have a dual style persona. The combination of which will give you a clearly designed roadmap to create your wardrobe successfully. Let's accept the skin we're in and the archetype and style persona that greets us in the mirror every morning.

Through the decades many consultants and stylists have attempted to create other descriptions for our bone structure and form. I am sticking to the original, ladies. If it isn't broken, don't fix it!

The 4 Classic Body Types are pretty self-explanatory: "H," "A," "8," and "V." No matter how much weight we gain or lose, our body type remains the same. Once we understand our basic body type, we can learn how to work our visual magic on our frame and create our own visual grammar and unique style.

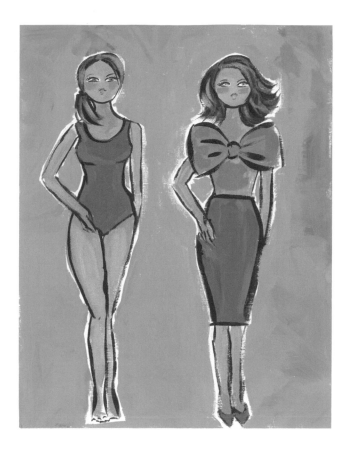

## "A" Frame

### The Ecstasy

The "A" frame is the most common body type. The great news about this figure type is that it tends to portray a younger, more youthful appearance over time, if we can manage to keep it in shape. Graceful neck and shoulders and a pretty décolleté are great assets as well as a small waist. Most American designers cut for this figure type because it is the most common silhouette in the U.S.

### The Agony

Weight gain occurs in the hips, stomach, and upper thighs, and it clearly throws this youthful appearance quickly into an older, more matronly look. Once weight is gained, it is very hard to take off in those problem areas. "A'" body types are usually long-waisted, a feature that fashion loves to adorn. The problem occurs if her legs are disproportionately short and full.

### The "A" Frame Body:

- Shoulders and chest are narrower than the hip and upper thigh area, which is structurally wider, thus the name "A"

- Spine may be curved with a protruding derriere or there may appear to have no derriere at all—it is flat
- The torso may be longer and the legs may be proportionately shorter and sometimes heavier
- Bust is usually average to small, rarely large
- When weight is gained, the initial place it shows is in the upper thighs and the hips

**The Trompe-l'oeil**

The "A" frame achieves a visually balanced look by creating the illusion of a wider shoulder area. This can be achieved by choosing garments with shoulder pads, using color blocking, and opting for specific neckline choices that expand and highlight the décolleté as well as using pattern and sleeve detail to create mass. Choose necklines that are bateau, sweetheart, or off the shoulder.

The "A" frame woman also looks great in dresses that accentuate the small waist and bust and lay softly or prominently over the hips like a shirt waist, princess, A-line, or peplum dress. Dress length and pant contour is also very important to elongate the leg and minimize the imbalance torso to leg ratio. Wear brighter and more expansive colors on the top half to visually expand the shoulder and bust area. Baubles bangles, ruffles and embellishments should also be worn here. Narrow bottom pants give the illusion of a longer leg. Forget about pleated and palazzo pants, lest your hip area will start resembling the very name is carries.

Choosing a darker color for the bottom narrows and recedes the area visually. Jackets that end mid-hip are best. Hemlines vary with overall height. Typically, the skirt should end at the best part of your leg; hovering around the knee is the most flattering length. Empire waists may elongate the leg as well.

*Developing a style is learning to wardrobe the body we were born with in such a way that we maximize its appeal with color, angles, proportions, detailing, and design.*

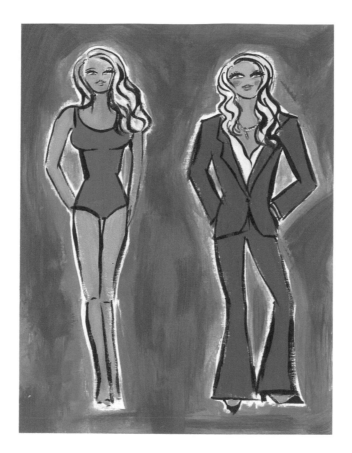

**"V" Frame**

### Ecstasy

I simply adore this shape! Wish I may, wish I might have this figure to flaunt tonight! It's so ironic how many women who sport this fabulous shape find themselves wishing they sported a different figure type. What are they thinking? So many world-class models find this figure to be an enormous asset when wearing clothes because the "V" body type is such a powerful image and anyone with this figure can own a room in a nanosecond! Great legs, amazing back, and a full bust? Where do I sign up?

### The Agony

Lots of ready-to-wear manufacturers do not cut for this figure, which can leave a girl very blue. As a child, many girls are criticized for their great shoulder and back. The linebacker references sting long after high school ends. Tsk! Tsk! Baby, look at you now!

### The "V" Frame Body

- Shoulders are visually wider than the hips
- Back is broader across the shoulders and architectural in shape
- Bust is usually larger with shorter waist. Occasionally small-busted women with an athletic build fit into this category.

*The "V" frame figure achieves balance by visually expanding the hip area and... visually lengthening the leg.*

- High, narrow hips and longer legs
- No true waist, rather a descending narrowness from shoulder to hip
- Derriere is usually flat
- Legs are normally long and thin and are considered to be a great feature
- Tummy can be flat or may become more prominent over time
- Initial weight gain is in the upper torso area

**The Trompe-l'oeil**

The "V" frame figure achieves balance by visually expanding the hip area and accentuating and visually lengthening the leg. This can be achieved with fabric choice, which can add volume to the hip, as well as using color blocking, which draws attention away from the shoulder and back and settles the eye on the legs and torso. Color choice, hip fabric fullness, the juxtaposition of patterned bottoms against a solid colored top, and wearing overblouses that lengthen the torso area are all great tricks. For those who can, wearing deep open backs, showing off their athletic build and body con clothing, which can accentuate their fabulous angularity, truly can set them apart from the rest!

"V" figures look absolutely fabulous in narrow slacks and tight jeans with a great blouse worn over the slacks—especially a well-fitting man-tailored shirt in a beautiful silk crepe or starched cotton. The open collar shows off their cleavage and the narrow leg accentuates their sporty powerful presence. Great-fitting luxe T-shirts have the same effect and can convey a more youthful image. At times, the bustline throws the whole figure way out of balance, and so separates tend to work better than dresses.

For those who do not have the bustline to carry the man's dress shirt off, I suggest knit tops that wrap the body totally around the viewer's eye, accentuating the overall shape, without noting the bustline at all.

Dresses can look fantastic as well. Add more fabric to the skirt to achieve balance with the top. Color blocking can visually narrow the shoulder area. Sleeves should be cut close to the body. Sleeveless is a great option for a woman who has toned arms, regardless of age.

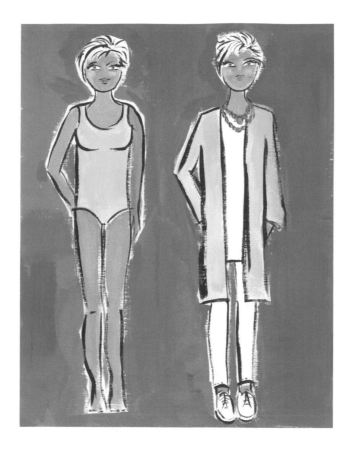

## "H" Frame

### The Ecstasy
Your legs are a great asset. Flaunt them, girls! The shoulders and hips are usually balanced, which makes the whole package look great! If weight is maintained, there is an overall visual balance that is lovely to look at and easy to wardrobe.

### The Agony
The plight of every "H" framed women is the fact that she has no waist to call her own. Many women try to compensate for this figure fact by insisting on wearing a belt or some waist-defining style to pretend to have one. This tactic is a disaster! The only thing that is achieved by creating a waist on a gal who doesn't have one is giving the impression that she has a fat waist. NOOOOO! The key to achieving balance in this situation is to ignore the waist area altogether. Camouflage the obvious and, trust me, no one will ever know that you don't have one.

### The "H" Frame Body
- Body is visually straight up and down without a clearly defined waist
- Shoulders and hips are balanced
- Thighs and derriere are usually flat

- Legs may be longer and usually thin
- Bust may be average to larger
- Waist is thicker
- Initial weight gain appears through the middle. The midriff, waist and tummy expand before the thighs and lower hips.

**The Trompe-l'oeil**

The H-Frame achieves figure balance by creating the illusion of a smaller waist by disguising it and distracting the viewer's eye to a prettier feature. The key is to define the smaller areas above or below the waist. The chemise or sheath dress works well as does a dress with an empire waist and straight drop. The BoHo look work well.

Another option is to create an outfit with slacks and a sweater set. Opt to wear either a longer open jacket like sweater straight or asymmetrical and a tank underneath, which gives the illusion of a waist. Color blocking and monochromatic styles work beautifully. Create vertical columns with your colors and designs that carry the eye from the shoulder to the leg (or longer) in a rectangular or triangular shape. The fabric separation does wonders! It alludes to a waistline that may be a bit broader than we would prefer. Overblouses with pretty necklines and prints also achieve the same effect as do over sweaters with a stylish faux dress shirt peeking through from the collar and tails. The contrasting collar and shirt tails distract the eye from the waist, and matching the sweater body with the slacks will elongate the torso.

*The plight of every "H" framed women is the fact that she has no waist to call her own... The key to achieving balance in this situation is to ignore the waist area altogether. Camouflage the obvious and, trust me, no one will ever know that you don't have one.*

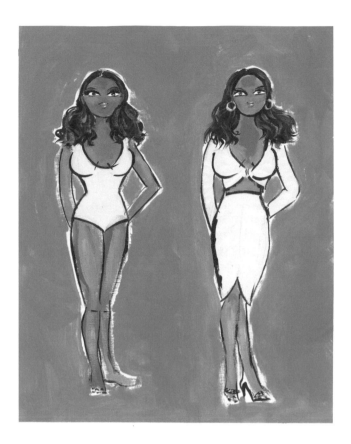

## "8" Frame

### The Ecstasy

This is a body many women want and men adore. She has that gorgeous, sexy hourglass shape that is defined and ever-present, boasting curves in all the right places and a fantastic waistline in between. Many film and TV stars rock this spectacular figure. The Figure 8 fills the dress with finesse, femininity, and pizzazz. Everyone's heads will turn when she enters a room, but being taken seriously and getting the response deserved may take some effort.

### The Agony

Not everyone can imagine what it's like to fit that glorious form into most ready-to-wear! Hourglass shaped women are subjected to a lot of dressing room humiliation and defeat, looking fab in bathing suits and clothes that are body conscious but disastrous in the rest. The good news: weight gain is in proportion. No matter her size, her body is fantastic. The bad news is that finding clothes can be a nightmare at any size.

### The "8" Frame Body
- Body is curvy and perfectly balanced
- Bust is full; waist is small and sometimes high

- Hips are fuller with a gentle taper and a nicely proportioned derriere
- Legs are generally curvy and thighs a bit full
- Leg length is in balance with torso
- Initial weight gain is evenly distributed throughout the body
- Beautiful décolleté
- Ultra-feminine mystique

**The Trompe-l'oeil**

The "8" frame is balanced and best shown off by accentuating the waistline. Avoid visual clutter such as layers and all-over patterns. Choose garments that naturally fit the body and move fluidly. Too much detail and embellishments are heavy and unflattering. Feminine, YES! Baby doll, NO!

The key to dressing success for an "8" is buying clothes that are cut curvy with rounded lines and shapes. Avoid straight lines and angularity altogether. The necklines are best round, sweetheart, off the shoulder, and scoop. Beware of showing off too much cleavage during the day. Wear undergarments that truly lift and separate. In addition, right shape wear will define your waist and smooth your hips. Knit dresses that that gently embrace your shape work beautifully. Lighter weights and softness work well as do medium to lighter weight knits and synthetics. Peplums look fabulous as do shorter fitted jackets with a lapelled collar and curved lines.

Slacks should be tapered and flat front. Too many pleats and patterns will make an "8" look frumpy and old. Less is more for these incredible bodies. There is nothing to camouflage here. For an "8," it's all about not overwhelming the world with that unstoppable fabulous frame!

# Strip Tease

**Eye Candy or Soul Food?**

As we have seen, every body type has its pluses! Sometimes a girl gets a bit carried away with flaunting what she's got. I'm taking a moment here to pontificate from Mount Glam on the pitfalls of being "Eye Candy" and the benefits of being "Soul Food."

What is alluded to, partially unveiled, and hidden… teased and kept unseen… is always exponentially more powerful than what is exposed and seen. Let the imagination fill in the nuances of your wardrobe against your skin. Seduction and allure lie in your silhouette. Keep a little mystery. Add a little mischief, and remain a bit enigmatic in your smile and your seams.

*Seduction and allure*
*lie in your silhouette.*
*Keep a little mystery.*
*Add a little mischief,*
*and remain a bit enigmatic*
*in your smile*
*and your seams.*

When selecting a garment, show off the best part of any single feature...and leave the rest for the chase. Every leg has a beautiful aspect. Find it. Define it. Flaunt it!

Once, a certain younger gentleman described to me how enticing it was to walk behind me, watching my wrap dress caress my thighs and derriere. He said the knee-length wrap revealed a graceful, elegant leg. He went on to confess that he couldn't stop thinking about what the rest of it might look like. I was astonished and amazed. Blushing and amused, I thought to myself, How do you like that! I never get these types of compliments wearing a thigh-high mini! This elegant, rather conservative guy taught me a huge lesson. Men love the hunt. They don't want you served up on a silver platter for all to see. Who says you can't learn a little from a young cub?

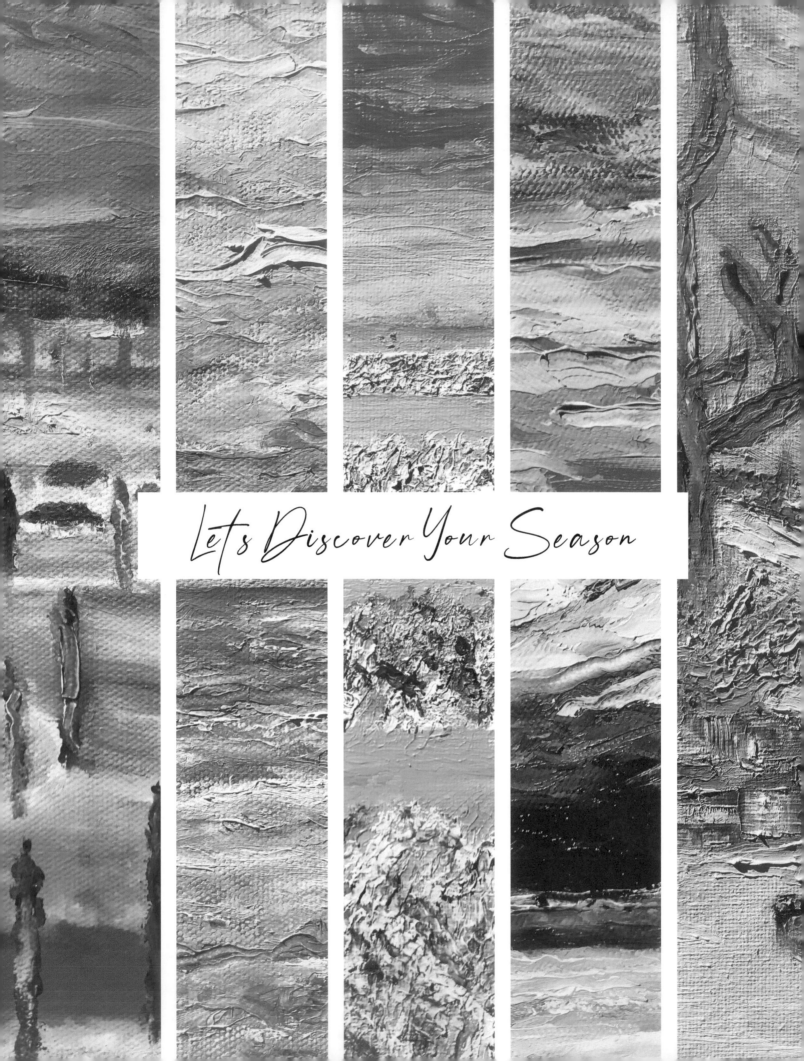

Let's Discover Your Season

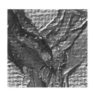

# CHAPTER 24

## Loving the Skin You're In

Did you know that wearing the right shades of color can actually make you look more energetic, younger, slimmer, successful, and attractive? Did you know that each of us has a base undertone to our skin that will determine the correct colors for you to wear in order for you to look your best?

This exciting color concept is not new. It is as relevant today as it was in 1980 when Carole Jackson wrote the book Color Me Beautiful. I have incorporated some of this system into my own work for over thirty years and use it every single day with my personal clients, worldwide, to ensure that the colors they wear will create a dynamic presence both on camera and in real life! Skin tone determines your best wardrobe colors and creates a younger, slimmer, sexier, and successful you!

**Am I Blue? Your Skin's Undertone**
Perhaps... or perhaps you are yellow. These are the two basic undertone colors. If your skin has a blue undertone, you are considered a "cool." If your skin has a yellow undertone, you are considered a "warm." The perfect shades of color for your wardrobe, hair, and makeup should have the same base undertone as your natural skin tone. Once we determine the correct skin tone, it is then important to further discover the "season" that best represents your skin's individual color personality.

Cool skin tones fall into "Winter" and "Summer." Approximately 80 percent of the population is Cool. Warm skin tones are divided into "Autumn" and "Spring." The explanation for this subdivision is quite simple: some skin tones look better in tints, tones, and shades of the pure chroma. Depending upon which variation suits you best, you will be considered to be typed as a "Season."

There is an even further delineation to determine the exact best color temperature for you: Light, True, and Vivid. A "Light Cool and Light Autumn" will look best in the lightest temperatures. A "Vivid" looks best in the hottest or brightest color saturation. A

*Skin tone determines your best wardrobe colors and creates a younger, slimmer, sexier, and successful you!*

"True" looks best in the middle ranges.

Once you determine whether you are a Cool or a Warm and then narrow yourself to a season and a temperature, you will have an exact palette to select your best colors.

A Hue is a color on the visible light spectrum based upon its wavelength. A Value is the lightness or darkness of a color.

Chroma is the quality of brightness or dullness of the color. Undertones are the colors you see when blue or yellow are added to the hue. They are the temperature of the color. Tints are pure hue with white added. Tones are pure hue with gray added. Shades are pure hue with black added. Every season can wear every color from the Visible Light Spectrum successfully, once it has been adjusted by value and chroma and undertone.

## Let's Discover Your Season!

Although it is not possible to be fully accurate in a virtual analysis, we can usually get pretty close to the truth. Here are your guidelines for discovering your Skin Season.

1.    Always look at yourself in natural daylight. Artificial light will camouflage your true skin color and make it very difficult to determine your true colors.
2.    Pull your hair back, so that it does not distract you in determining your skin undertone.
3.    Make sure that you have no makeup on while determining your colors.
4.    If you are having trouble deciding, ask a friend to help you.

**How to determine which shades look best:**

1.    Does this color make you look younger or older?
2.    Does this color make you look tired or energetic?
3.    Does this color make your teeth look white or yellow?
4.    Does this color make you look heavier or slimmer?
5.    Only compare the color against your skin tone. Do not consider your eyes or hair.

# Cool/Warm Analysis

**Choose one:**

**I look better in:**
1. Black
2. Brown

**I look better in:**
1. Silver
2. Gold

**I look better in:**
1. Pink
2. Orange

**I look better in:**
1. White
2. Cream

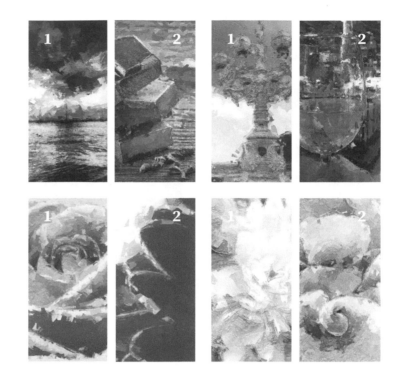

If your answers are mostly 1s, you are a Cool.
If your answers are mostly 2s, you are a Warm.

Now you have determined whether you are a Warm or a Cool. If you are a Cool, we now must decide if you are a Winter or Summer.

*Here are some hints to help you decide whether you are a Winter, Summer, Autumn, or Spring.*

# Winters often have:

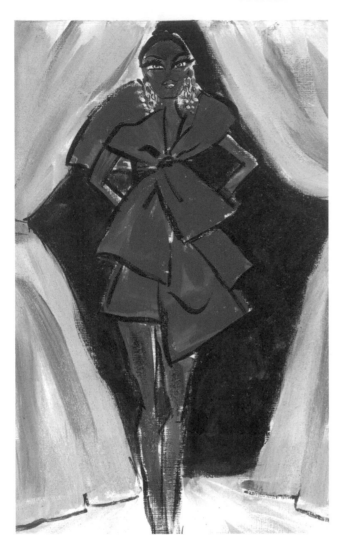

### Skin
- Pale, porcelain
- Pale or rosy beige
- Ruddy with red and pink tones
- Very dark brown or black
- Copper, or medium to dark browns of
- Honey browns or
- Olive tones or
- Peachy beige

### Natural Hair Color
- Darkest blacks and browns
- Silvery gray, tends to salt and pepper
- Medium and dark browns, and darkest blacks, or
- Silvery gray, tends to salt and pepper
- Light red to strawberry

### Eye Color
- Deep browns and hazels
- Cool browns
- Darker blues
- Gray greens
- Medium to dark vibrant browns
- Golden and green hazels

*Cool skin tones fall into "Winter" and "Summer." Warm skin tones are divided into "Autumn" and "Spring."*

## Summers often have:

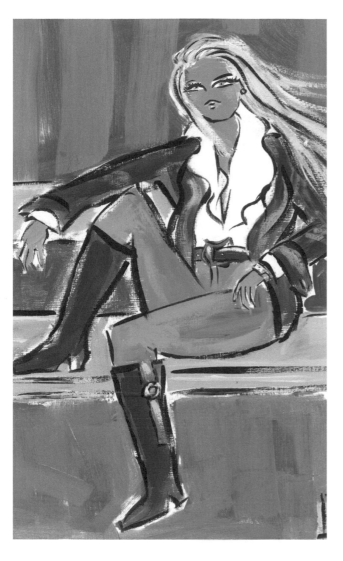

### Skin
- Very fair porcelain skin
- Pinkish or pinkish beige
- Ruddy (means reddish)
- Yellowish beige

### Natural Hair Color
- Ashy blondes and browns that tend to look dull and lifeless
- Gray and smoky blondes (platinum blonde as a child)
- Very dark brown
- Gray (ashy tones)

### Eye Color
- Any shade of blue
- Gray
- Gray-green and green with yellow radiating from the pupil or
- Hazel or gray-brown

*Once you determine whether you are a Cool or a Warm and then narrow yourself to a season and a temperature, you will have an exact palette to select your best colors.*

## Spring-toned people have a warm undertone, and have the following characteristics:

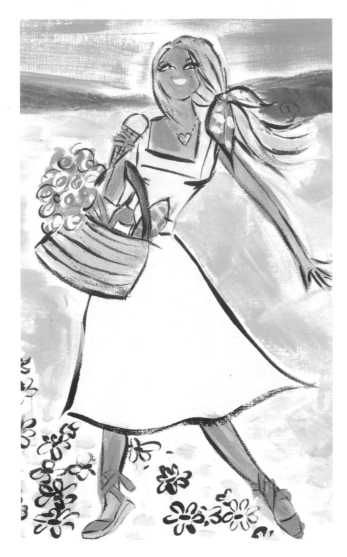

### Skin
- Ivory or milky white (can have freckles)
- Golden and peachy beige
- Ruddy with peach, pink or red tones

### Natural Hair Color
- Golden or honey blondes
- Strawberry blondes
- Reds and auburns
- Warm browns, occasionally dark brown, or
- Yellow-gray

### Eye Color
- Clear, light blues
- Any green shade
- Golden browns and hazels (not usually dark)

*The perfect shades of color for your wardrobe, hair, and makeup should have the same base undertone as your natural skin tone.*

## Autumns often have:

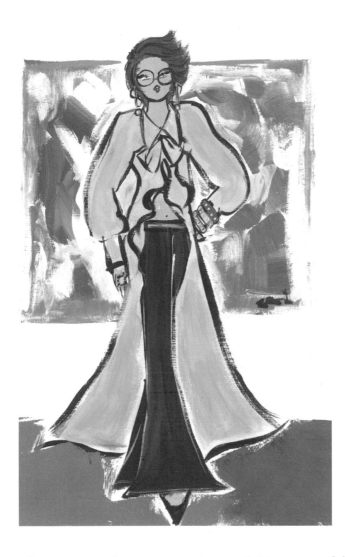

### Skin
- Ivory or light beige (can have freckles)
- Peachy or ruddy with peachy tones
- Golden beige or bronze

### Natural Hair Color
- Honey blondes
- Vibrant reds
- Reddish and coppery browns (medium to dark)
- Very black
- Yellowish gray

### Eye Color
- Dark to golden browns and hazels
- Green and blue hazels
- Dark or light greens
- Vibrant blues, never blue-gray

Now you have been able to determine whether you are a Cool or a Warm skin tone. Many of you will be able to further delineate whether you are a Summer, Winter, Spring, or Autumn.

Please go to the next session and discover which specific colors and palettes will make you look gorgeous and feel great!

*Did you know that wearing the right shades of color can actually make you look more energetic, younger, slimmer, successful, and attractive?*

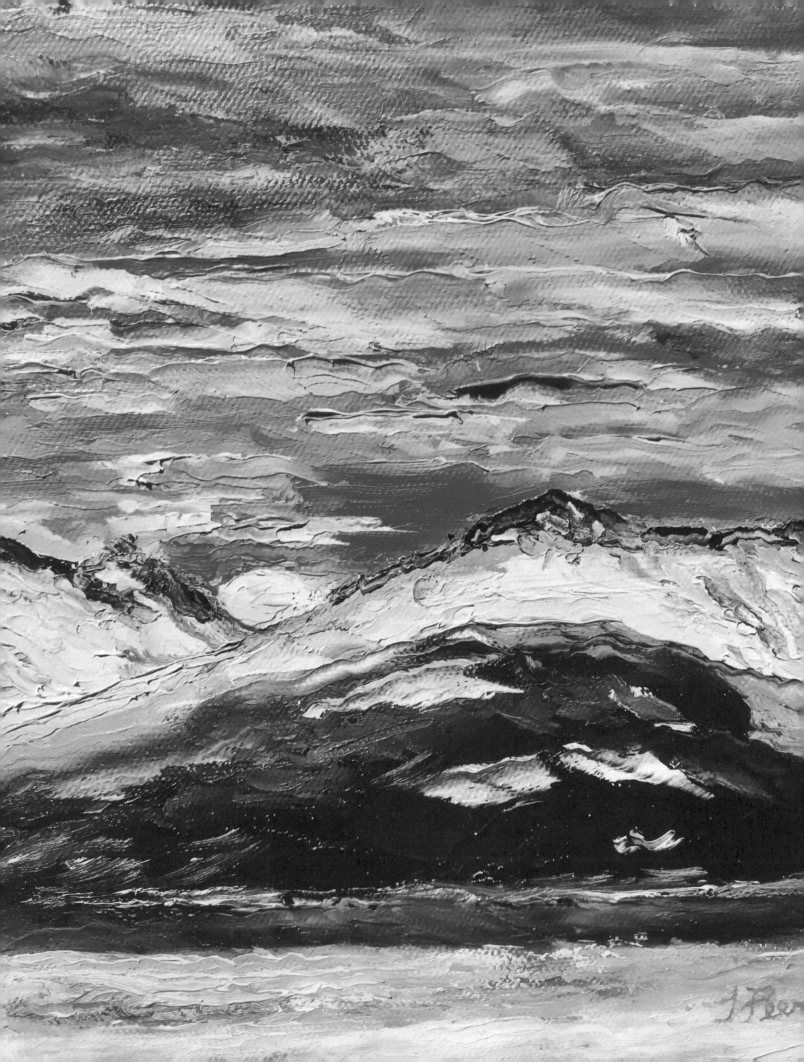

## Seasonal Palettes and You

Fantastic! We have your season selected. Now let's chat about the specific color palettes that will uplift and support your image and get you to the next level of success in your personal and professional relationships. The most important one being with you.

# Winter

Winters look great in the strongest color values possible and thrive in high contrasts. Think of the boldest and biggest colors. That is your palette. Think about a winter snowscape. Whether in the city or in the country, it offers stark contrasts that highlight the bold colors that thrive in shivering cold climates. Add the snow crystals and icicles and you will begin to understand the scope of your personal best colors for your wardrobe. Blacks, whites, steely grays, reds, shocking pinks, emerald greens, electric blues, and amethyst purples were made for you! Along with most of the neon and fluorescent colors that are so popular (fluorescent fabrics and lights have a natural blue undertone), your palette makes a bold and beautiful statement.

True Winters look best in these primary and secondary chroma, but the temperature of these shades should be a bit more toned down.

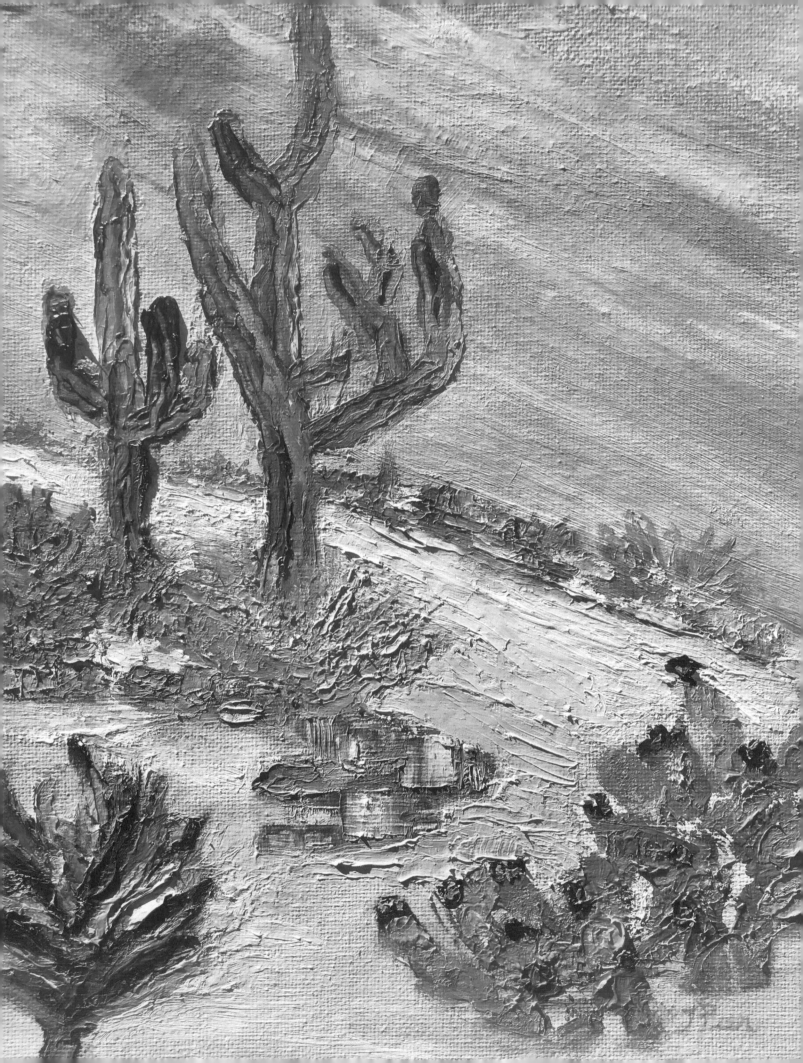

# Light Winter

Light Winters (Winter 2) look best in the lightest shades of these primary and secondary palettes, and many times they can wear shades that look great on Vivid Summers. Light Winters can be easily overpowered by high-voltage shades. A more muted and subtle palette will enhance their delicate coloring. The result will be fabulous.

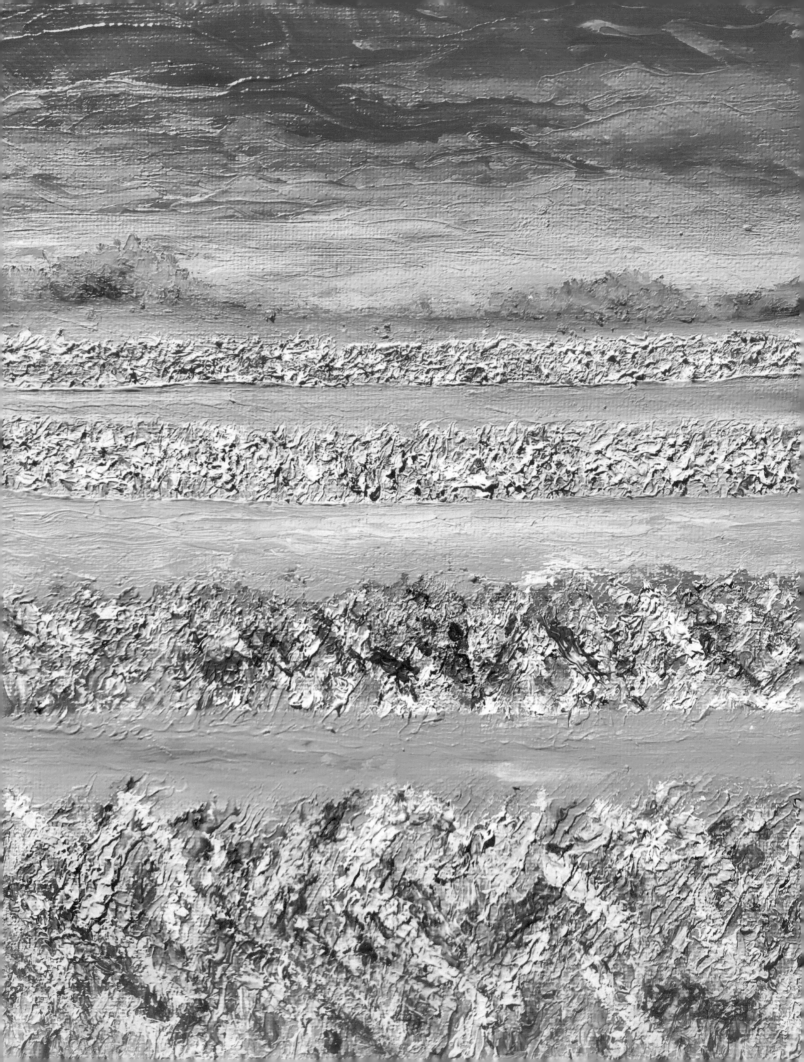

# Summer

Summers look best in pure chromes with gray added. In other words, they look terrific in misty morning shades whether beachside, countryside, mountainside, or cityscapes. More subtle hues with a touch of gray added make a Summer's complexion shine bright! Vivid Summers can wear the boldest temperatures in the palette. True Summers are straight down the center, and Light Summers look great in the lightest values of the Summer Palette.

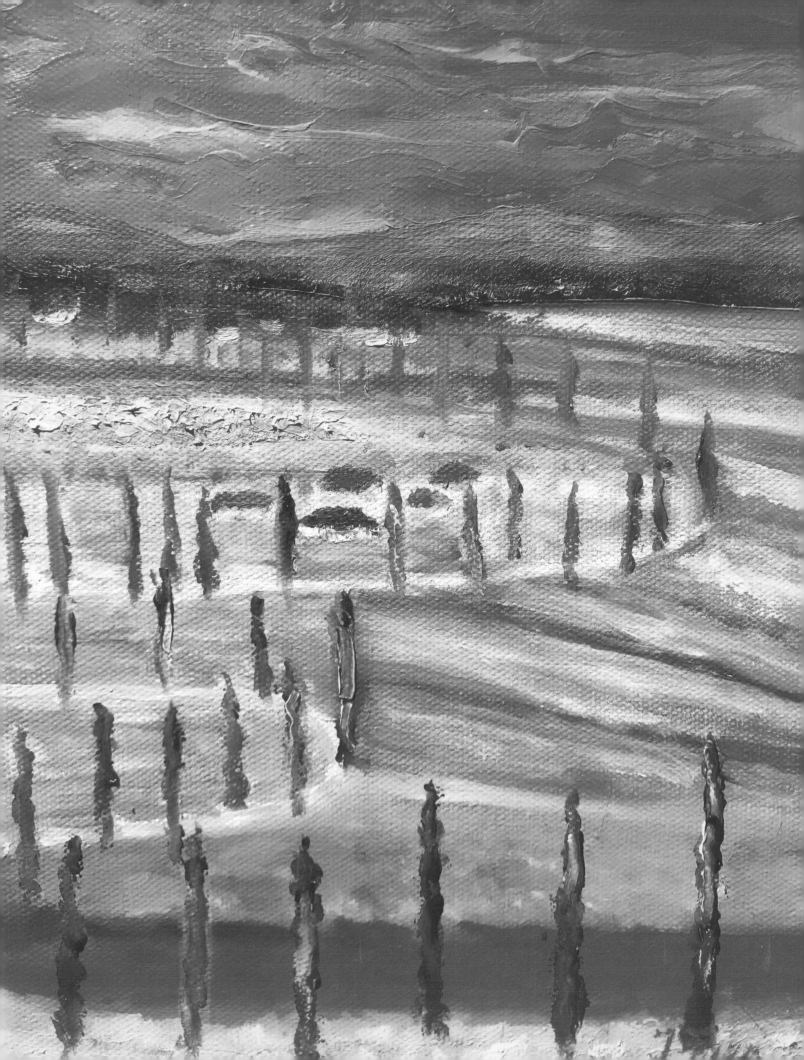

# Autumn

Autumn palettes also offer the richness and textures of fall in Vermont or anywhere the trees become ablaze with reds, oranges, golden yellows, and rich, earthy browns. Autumns embrace the gorgeousness and ruggedness of our national parks and exquisite heritage. Jewel tones will bring out the beauty and grace of the autumn personality. Vivid autumns wear the boldest and brightest jewel tones the very best. True Autumns look best in the medium values, and Light Autumns are best in the lighter temperature hues for the Autumn palette.

# Spring

Springs are the rarest season. Springs are the rarest complexions. They truly have a sparkle in their eye and a freshness to their complexion.

The Spring palette is best described by all the colors that represent Spring: Clear pastels of all temperatures work best for the pretty Spring persona. Think Easter eggs, jellybeans, tulips, and hyacinth...you get the picture. Vivid Springs can wear the hottest temperatures and many can also wear the lightest of the Autumn palettes as well, and vice versa. Medium Springs look great in mid-range tones, and Light Springs are made for the clearest and most delicate pastel colors.

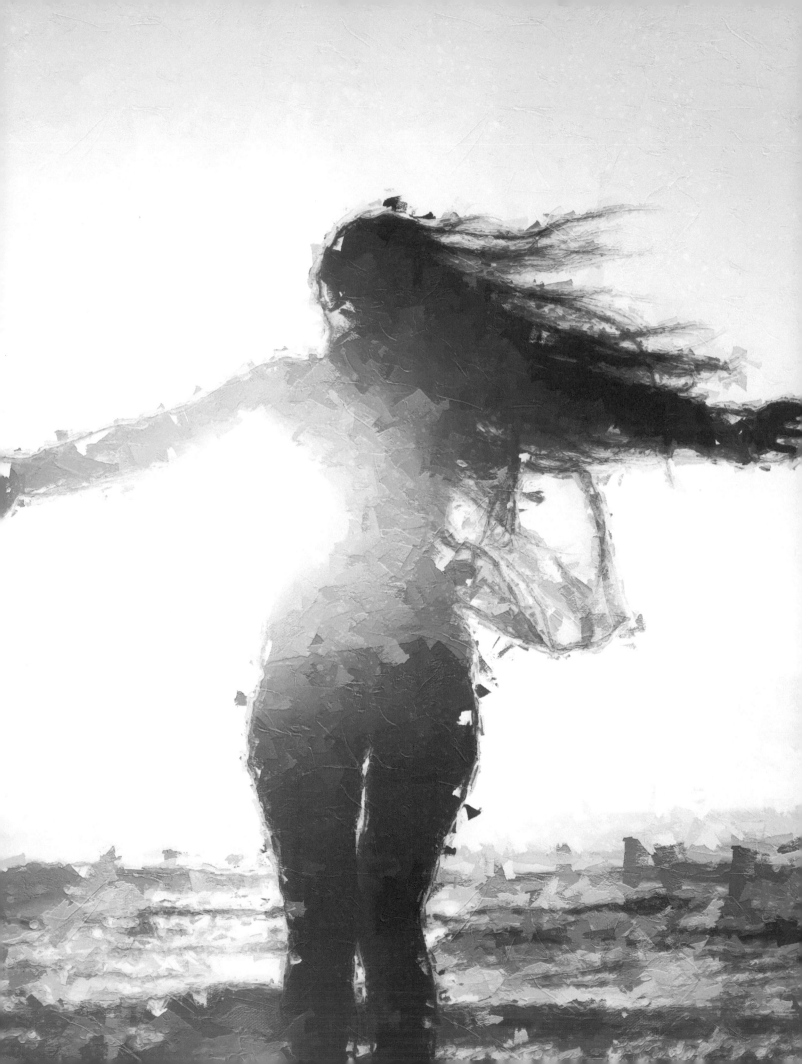

# CHAPTER 25
## *Your Divine Colors*

What if you had a language that spoke directly from your soul and created a rainbow that would describe and support your everyday life? Let me share this secret: You do! You possess a Divine Color Palette that will define who you are in a totally new and fascinating way, translate the world, and give you confidence, clarity, and self-compassion. It expresses your unique journey through the world in a way that makes perfect sense and allows you to understand yourself like never before. Success, happiness, love, and significance are waiting for you at the end of your rainbow. Welcome to the extraordinary world of color.

Your Divine Color Personality is as unique as your fingerprint. This unseen reality can be understood as a unique set of energetic hues that reflect and permeate every layer of your being. These extraordinary chromas create a vibration that goes beyond, taste, smell, touch, and hearing. These vibrations emit from deep within your soul, reflecting your true nature, your authentic self. Your unique color pattern, when in balance, provides you with a full spectrum of vibrational support, allowing you to not only feel secure and dynamic but actually contribute greatly to your communication to others and the entire world.

In addition to your personal palette, colors themselves possess certain inherent vibrational messages that convey emotional, intellectual, and physical information to others. These colors can support your internal environment and everyone else's too. Once you understand your own Divine Color Palette and Personality, the impact of color on others, and the dynamic role color plays in every human experience. Your relationships will be greatly enhanced. Your understanding of others will be clarified and your messages will be more clearly conveyed and received. Color will bring you success personally and professionally. You will have the tools to create great relationships and a happy and fulfilling life. Not only that, you will have a brand-new way to understand and communicate with your friends, loved ones, and coworkers.

> *"You possess a divine color palette that will define you in a new and totally fascinating way."*

How did I discover it? I have always had a passion for and an inherent understanding of color. My early memories are saturated with light and chroma. My childhood experiences were augmented and remembered in vivid hues and sounds.

When I was about four or five, I was sitting at the kitchen table before the light of day. Nana always rose way before the sun, busily preparing the most scrumptious baked goods for breakfast.... I couldn't miss a thing. During those wee hours we would discuss all the world's most important items especially all things beauty, art, and joy! She was a fashion designer by trade.

One morning, we were discussing a dress that I wanted her to make for me. She asked me about the color. I said, "I want a pink dress, Nana!" Then she asked what shade of pink. Embarrassed, quite taken aback, and having no concrete language for the color in my mind's eye, I decided that that was never going to happen again. I asked my Mom for a huge box of crayons and spent the next week memorizing all the colors and their names. The next time Nana asked me about a shade of pink, I was very proud to share my knowledge. "Let's make it cameo, or should it be fuchsia or carnation?" Yes, I had memorized every single color, becoming fluent in the language, ready to put it to good use. That childhood experience was the beginning of my love affair with color.

Decades later, on board a ship cruising the Mediterranean with my Mom and kids, the universe dropped this extraordinary understanding of vibrational color and healing right into my lap. I knew immediately that this expertise and deep awareness was way beyond the norm. I realized my ability to channel color was given to me to share with the world. Since that day, I have worked with thousands of people in the discovery and implementation of their Divine Color Palette. I have done television, radio, lectures, and classes, and now it's time to bring the divine world of color into focus for you!

What is your favorite color? Don't think about it for too long. Write down your favorite color or two colors at most. What was your favorite color as a child? These are not necessarily the colors that look good on you. These are simply colors that exist in the world that you like and, for many of you, have always liked. Now write down the color you dislike the most. They are a crystal ball revealing your inner truths and biases as well as your personality.

For now, we are going to chat about color in general terms. Your favorite colors, especially your childhood favorites, speak volumes about your authentic self, revealing the qualities given to you at birth. Many factors contribute to creating your soul's palette. Life experience can alter perceptions and feelings about colors. This mini exploration will give you an initial insight and understanding of your color affinity.

The following descriptions can be used as a general guideline for selecting color schemes for your personal and professional life: wardrobe, home and office decor and designs, branding, marketing, even entertaining. If you are interested in discovering your color personality in great depth, and I suggest you do, you might consider a private consultation. It will change your life.

## Colors and Their Vibrational Meanings, Psychological Impacts, and Emotional Overlays

Let's explore each Divine Color Personality and its attributes. Please keep in mind that this is a general overview. Once you identify your unique color palette, it will be easy to create a wardrobe that conveys familiarity, relatability, likability, relevance, and confidence. Color vibration creates nonverbal attraction and affinity.

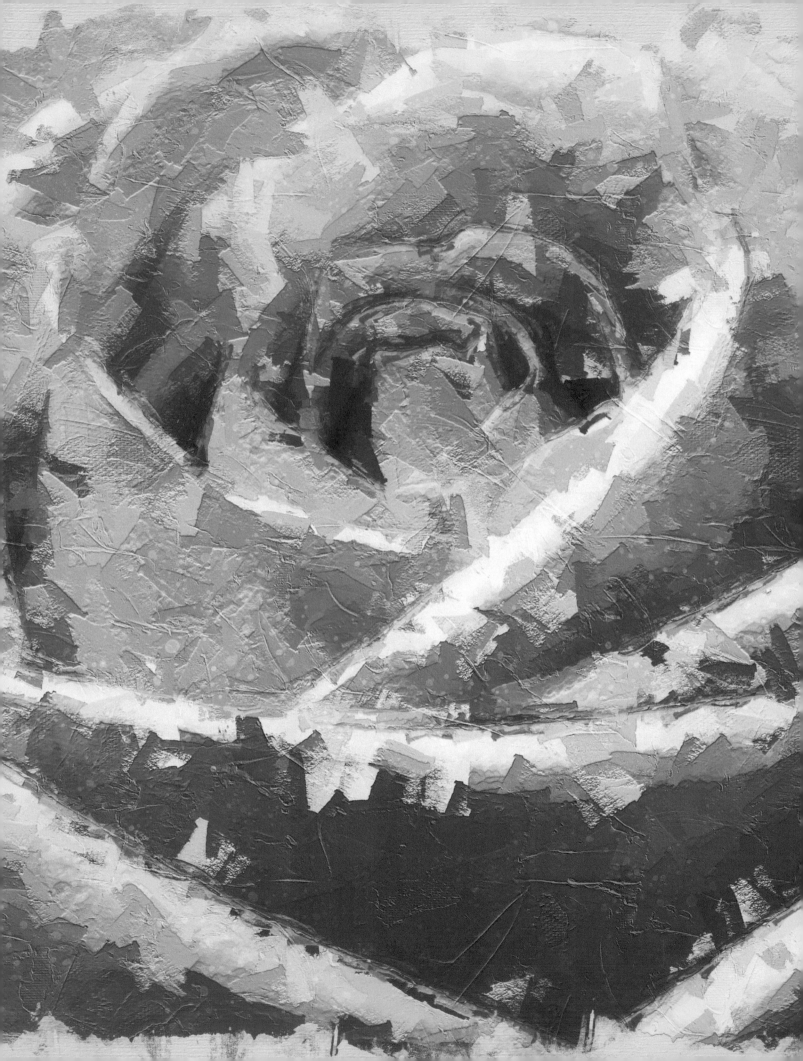

# Pink

Pink is the color of love. Love for self, love for others, and love for the Divine. Pink girls are love incarnate. They love every living thing without hesitation or judgment. They give hugs to the planet in large ways and small, and rarely have boundaries or expectations for anything in return. Pinks process their world emotionally first. They are highly intuitive and trust their inner guidance system to lead the way. They love entirely and immediately. They are compassionate and all-consuming.

Pink personalities lead with the heart, trusting its knowledge in all matters. They make decisions based upon instinct. Emotions guide their journey. This is the good and the sometimes painful news. Pinks love. Period. Once a pink discovers and embraces their own capacity to love fully and freely, they know "who" they are in the world. Significance begins and ends with love. It is their raison d'être. Pinks are the lovers of this planet, and because of this extraordinary quality, they are also great healers and nurturers.

Pinks facilitate discovering love in others, establish love connections, experience empathy, and connect hearts. Their skills are used to facilitate very vulnerable and deeply personal explorations with heart-centered listening, and see loving essence while reflecting and exploring feelings. Pinks provide the foundation for all the other colors to manifest and actualize at their highest and best. It is the soul. Without true understanding of love, compassion, and empathy, there is no hope for relationships, growth, integration, or self-actualization. Love truly does make the world go around.

## The Divine Color of LOVE

# Red

Red is the color of passion, action, sexuality, physicality, and Chi. It is a fight or flight color. which actually raises blood pressure and immediately viscerally affects those who are visually engaged. Reds are "Get on my jet or get off my runway" kind of women! These women are expansive personalities, relentlessly in pursuit of whatever it is they want to own, do, or achieve. They are powerhouses. They are natural-born leaders possessing strong egos and opinions. You will intimately know them both! Red women rule their universe. They process the world physically first. Act now… think and feel later.… They are the take-action souls of the Divine Color Palette, transforming themselves and the world.

Red personalities are the "movers and shakers" of the planet. They are quick, decisive, and candid, living fast and furious, making instant decisions, having things their way and leaving the mess for someone else to address! They are risk takers and bore easily. Reds manifest their desires at any cost.

Focus, energy, and enthusiasm fuel their fire. In order for a Red woman to enjoy a healthy, joy-filled life, she must get down to the very essence of what motivates her to act and accomplish her goals. Right or wrong, passion leads the way. Reds get things done by putting plans into action, often weighing their own worth and value by their achievements and accumulating accolades and possessions. This brings a sense of happiness and fulfillment.

## *The Divine Color of PASSION and ACTION*

# Blue

Blue is the color of trust, integrity, high mental serenity, intellect, and loyalty. It is America's number one favorite color. Blue personalities are extremely loyal, integrous, and diligent to the point of perfectionism. She works best as a support person and team player. She is very happy in a support position either in a relationship or a career, not needing the ego satisfaction of taking the lead, but truly capable of being the star of the show. Blue gals process the world mentally first. If things make sense, then they are more likely to emotionally and physically engage in relationships, choices, and situations.

Blue personalities are diplomatic, conscientious, and caring. They are team players, providing tremendous support and leadership without wanting or needing to receive recognition or attention. Blue women are practical thinkers, taking a methodical approach to problem solving and establishing order from chaos. They care and love deeply and make tremendous partners and parents.

Blues use their high mental capacity to navigate their lives one step at a time. They are often given tremendous responsibility and are 100 percent responsible for their actions and their behavior. A Blue woman's integrity and reputation are extremely important to her. Decisions are careful, and predictive, safe outcomes are highly desirable. They are diplomatic and slow to anger. Moral values, intuition, conscience, goal-setting ability, and productivity are all wrapped up in Miss Blue! She is the "Big Picture" gal providing rational thought and practical sense to everyday life.

## The Divine Color of
## HIGHER INTELLECT
## and MENTAL SERENITY

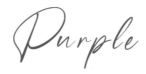

# Purple

Purple is the color of creativity, spirituality, and forgiveness. It ranks high in likability for women. Purple Personalities are unique in all the world. They say it like they see it... long on candor, often short on tact. They mean no harm. Their perspective on life is totally unique and their lifestyle choices often reflect their individuality, spirituality, and creativity.

Purples cha-cha to the beat of their own drum...needing to relate to other purples to establish a true mind meld. Purple is a combination of red and blue. Honest and frank, they see it, think about it, say it, and do it. Purple women do not have a filter. Depending upon the other colors in their palette, these extraordinary women delve deeply into one or two branches of their tree... spiritually, creativity, or forgiveness. From psychologist to healer, Purple women offer a unique perspective and creative approach to living.

Purple personalities are purple through and through! They are extremely original in their thoughts, actions, and self-creation. They tend to be an odd blend of highly spirituality and extreme practicality. Very individualistic and somewhat opinionated, they are often misunderstood because their best intentions and actions do not always translate to others with the goodness and care they embody.

Purples are very spiritual, even psychic. Their connection to the Divine is instant and absolute. They manifest their lives the best they can, often in spite of their huge imaginations. Many purples live two lives: the ones the world sees and the private world they create for themselves and/or channel from other dimensions. Virtual reality is no stranger to these extraordinary, unconventional, and extremely capable beings.

Because of their truly unique understating and perspective, Purples often process the world through their third eye. They are creatives regardless of their job title. Purple women stick together. They understand each other and seek refuge from the world away from those who don't get them. Purples are transformational and spirit-filled. Faith, courage, and fortitude are all housed here. They express acceptance and self-forgiveness as well as facilitating forgiveness in others.

## The Divine Color of CREATIVITY, SPIRITUALITY and FORGIVENESS

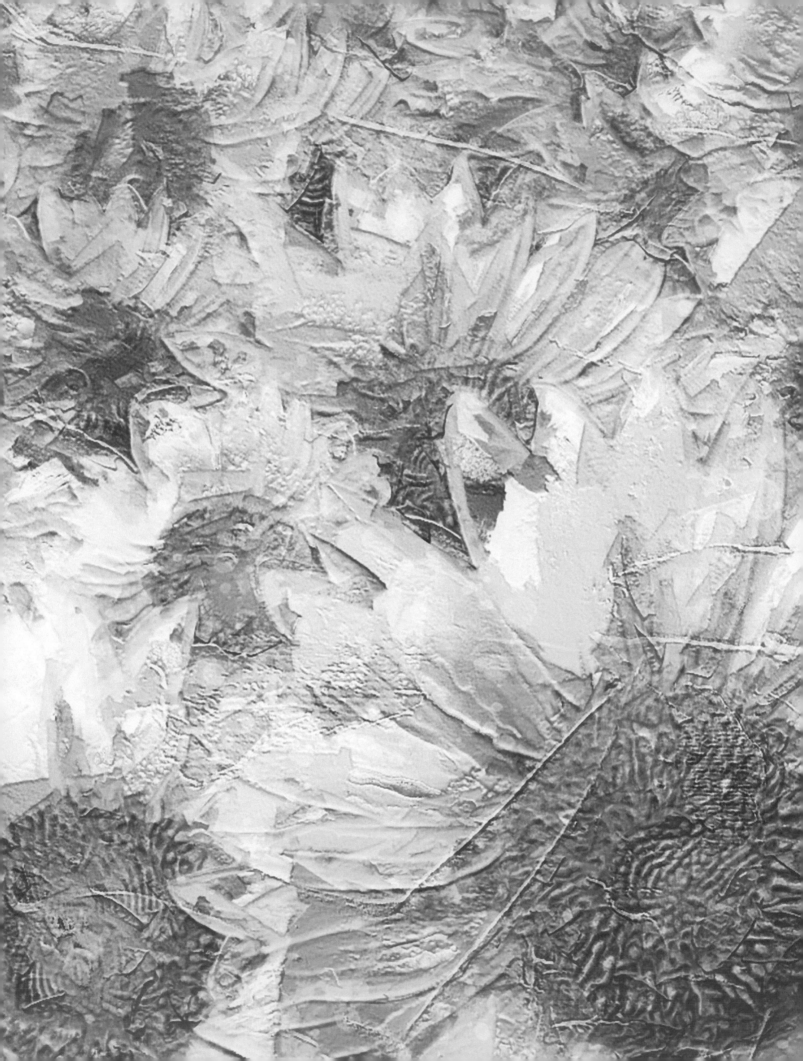

Yellow is the color of mental clarity and optimism. It forces the eye and brain to focus on a task. Yellows are hardly mellow. Possessing keen mental acuity and a heightened sense of focus, these analytical gals are quick-thinking, problem-solving, intellectual forces to be reckoned with. They also process the world mentally first...they are passionate about resolving conflicts and solving problems in an innovative and unique way. The sunshiny news is that Yellow women have the answer... even if you didn't realize that you have a question! Their optimism stems from their mental inquisitiveness and utter confidence. They pack hope and happiness in their toolbox and a spreadsheet too!

Yellow personalities make sense of the world in a very logical methodical without establishing an emotional connection. Yellow personas do not internalize feelings the same way other colors do. That is not to say that Yellow personalities are unfeeling. Yellow personas do feel. Eventually... if it makes sense... and if they can find the pathway to their heart. These women need to impose order in the world. They deal in the facts and have no interest or trust in emotions to create a meaningful life. They create a plan with concentration and clarity and then apply the focus and determination to execute it effectively.

Yellow personalities are optimistic and decisive, maximizing brain power, clearing out the cobwebs, and directing joy like a laser beam! They are awake and enjoy sharing their observations and insights with others in order to better lives and the planet!

These women supply hard drives for our world. Information is power and joy. Control over information and figuring out the answers to complex issues and problems are what they love to do. They measure everything in life. Everything and everyone must make sense, have a purpose, and fill a need without costing too much. Yellows are organized and pragmatic. They are laser sharp and like to have concrete, finite solutions.

Yellow personalities are skeptical by nature but generally very positive people. They are pleasant to be around and easy to get along with except where facts and figures are concerned. They are very precise in all they do. Cleanliness is orderliness, and order is heavenly. They are not interested in breaking the mold for their lives. They enjoy knowing how their life will play out and are not interested in surprises or risks unless highly calculated in their favor. They are the mathematicians of our world. Black and white makes sunshine for yellow personas.

*The Divine Color of MENTAL CLARITY, POSITIVITY and HOPE*

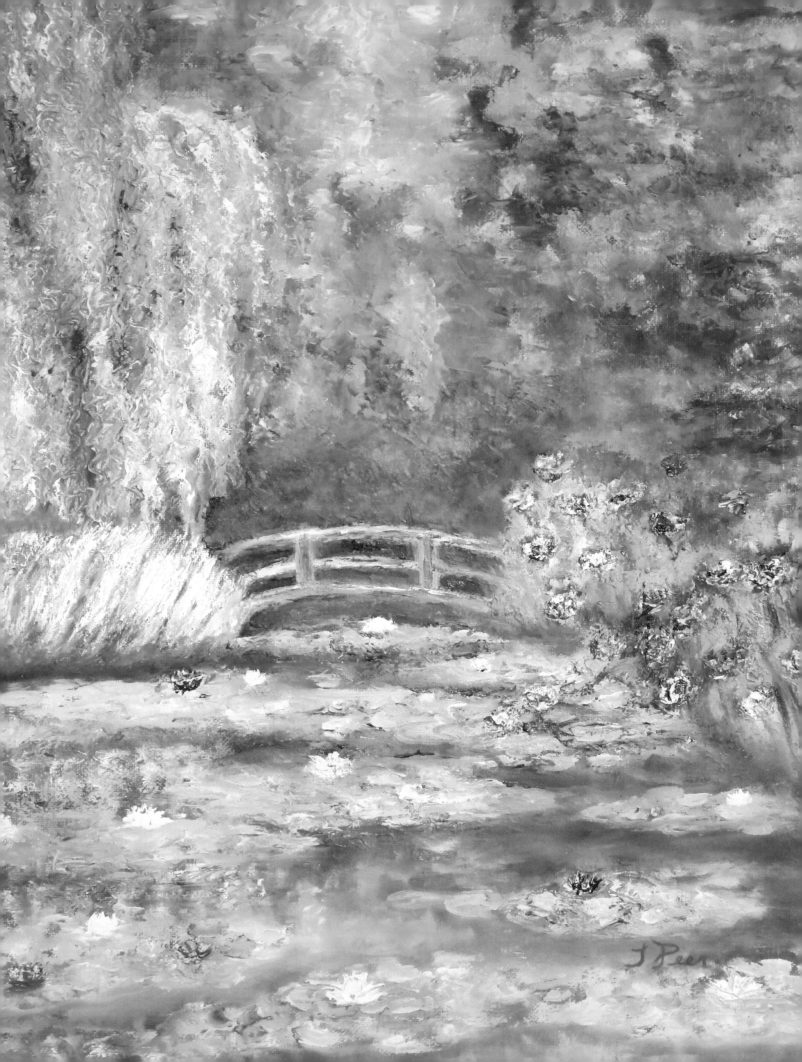

# *Turquoise*

Turquoise is the color of communication. Its fresh green influence refreshes and energizes the vibrational field. Once combined with all the mental energy and integrity of blue and the mental clarity and positivity of yellow, this spectacular color is alluring and captivating for the observer and uplifting and inspiring for the wearer as well. Turquoise creates an immediate rapport between people, providing a gateway for open conversation and collaboration. Turquoise ladies are very bright and have a twinkle in their eyes. They are blessed with the gift of gab and happy to share it with the world. Often asked to speak, they are able to lightheartedly and accurately describe any situation with humor and enthusiasm. No wonder so many TV personalities are attracted to this hue.

Turquoises are the planet's communicators. They harness their emotions, thoughts, and energy into creating and conveying ideas to others in a dynamic and engaging way. Magnetic and articulate, these cool beauties are natural connectors, speakers, broadcasters, and persuaders, possessing style, skill, and savvy. Turquoise women are the bridge-makers of our society, often bringing people together in a way that fosters kindness and understanding, solutions, epiphanies, and self-expression. They have a highly developed soft skill set as well as a natural way to transmit ideas and feelings in a most entertaining, enlightening, and educational way. A message has no value unless it is being clearly sent and received. Turquoises express opinions in order to achieve goals as well as gaining consensus. They provide society with a power assist in achieving understanding and fulfillment. Their ability to communicate effectively allows them to influence others and educate the planet.

## *The Divine Color of COMMUNICATION*

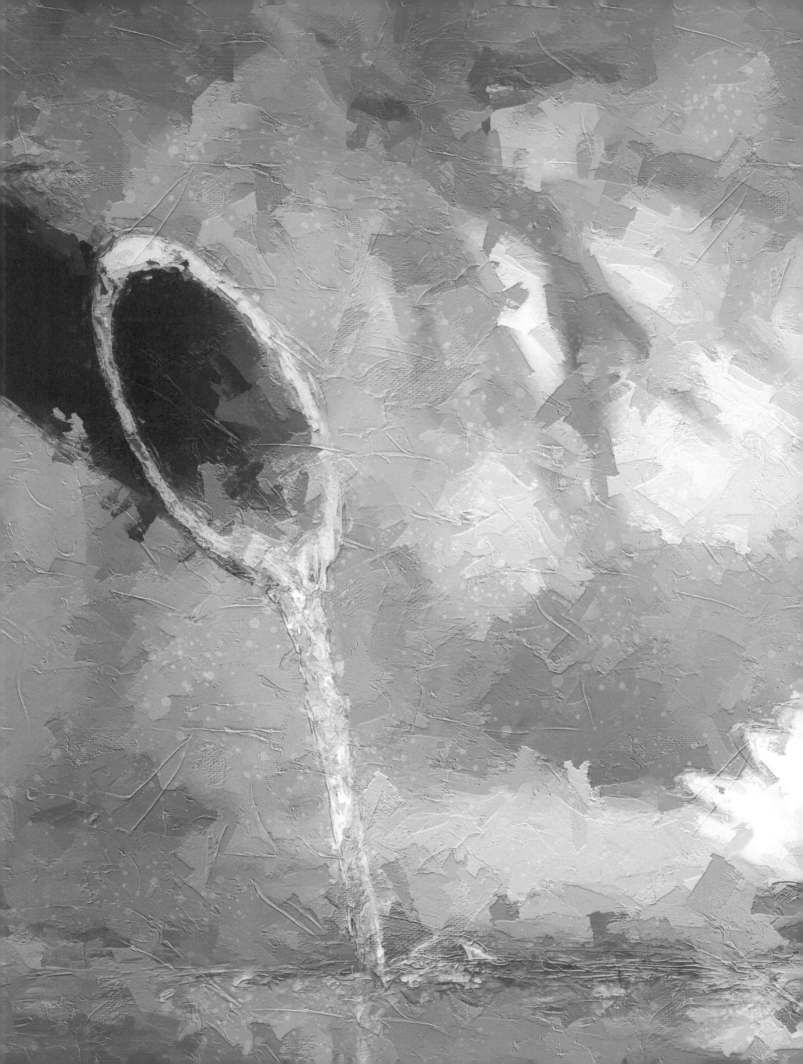

# Green

Green is the color of balance, peace, nature, conviviality, and volunteerism. What Green personalities want most is to live in peace and serenity. They sacrifice personally to establish calm and conviviality wherever they spend their time. Greens are the "do-gooders" of the planet. Their joy and happiness come from doing and being in a state of fairness, balance, order, and comradery. They put their money and time where their mouth is: They don't just think about doing good... they do good in life and in their careers. Greens have a strong sensibility and need for being close to nature, and they rely on these moments to re-energize, restore, and replenish themselves.

More than any other color personality, Greens strive to create peace and balance in the world at large and oftentimes sacrifice their own goals and desires in order to avoid problems and arguments personally and professionally. Green women provide a shoulder to lean on, a helping hand and a warm smile to anyone who needs it, using their gifts and talents to promote health, vitality, and harmony. They also provide care to those in need. Very aware of the power of nature and inspired by its beauty, Green personalities spend time in the outdoors and care about environmental issues and social causes. They do not have to be right all the time, truly embodying an ego that is balanced and stays in check. Greens just want everyone to get along and be happy.

Greens are generous and sociable. They are activists and good neighbors. They are like seesaws seeking homeostasis, relaxation and restoration. Green is the conduit for consistency and calmness. The healing qualities of the green vibration provides an internal connection to the natural path of life. They provide a spiritual, mental, and physical detox for the world and promote living stress free and within the natural order.

## The Divine Color of
## BALANCE AND PEACE

# White

White is the heavenly color embodying the perfect balance of all the vibrational colors in the visible spectrum. It is the color of divinity. White signifies a higher consciousness, divine inspiration and enlightenment. This vibration is achieved through living a highest and best life. White is also the color of purity, not in the sense of innocence, but rather in the sense of wisdom gained through years of dedication, devotion, and understanding. The higher consciousness resonates in this hue, and those who are attracted to it are "full in" on their journey with destiny.

They possess a certain calmness that is truly Zen. Their spirituality is all present and fully immersive. White can become a very isolating and unsettling color for some. It is demanding in its solitude and relentless in its ability to see right through to the essence of one's soul. White personalities are transformationalists and, often, openly share their connection with the universe.

White is the culmination and combination of all color. It clearly embraces connection to the Divine—whatever that means to the individual. White personalities usually develop over years of enlightenment and transformational work. They have walked the walk and talked the talk. They have prayed, meditated, journeyed, loved, forgiven, and somewhere along the line become wiser and accepting of the Divine nature and symmetry of human existence. White personalities have a knowingness that transcends knowledge and an ability to remain pure and open to beings with as little filter and bias as humanly possible. This does not mean that white personalities are saints... it just means that they have worked on themselves extensively and have arrived at a juncture that incorporates all the other colors into their energy field with harmony and balance.

White personalities are a bit enigmatic... perhaps a bit removed. Often by choice. They are strong, powerful, and fully aware that the potential emanating from them is not their own. They will always carry the essence of their original Divine Color Palette and, quite often, will have another favorite along with white. White personalities have grown comfortable in their own skin... the spectrum provides the inner cleansing, childlike laughter, and wonder necessary for a joy-filled life.

## *The Divine Color of DIVINITY, ENLIGHTENMENT, PURITY and CONFIDENCE*

# Beige

Beige signifies neutrality and impartiality, creating a level playing field and a non-judgmental environment for providing conversation, discussion, problem solving, and cooperative communication. Beige personalities are tactful and honest, gracious and patient in their demeanor. Their strength lies in their ability to create a platform that is non-critical and fair. Beige women have the ability to arbitrate with confidence and tact, providing space and understanding for all sides of a dispute so that conflict resolution can be attained.

Beige personalities are experts in "holding space" for others to ventilate their thoughts and emotions and come to terms with their feelings so that a positive outcome can be achieved for all concerned. They are extremely clear and very grounded in their approach to life and an asset to any volatile situation. Beige women also embody the undertones of whatever the base shade exists in the chroma.

Beige personas are highly respected and admired for a calm and elegant persona. They exude confidence and collectivism in all situations, guided by reason and moderation. Beiges have the highly sought-after ability to remain neutral in emotionally charged situations. They offer sage advice and sound judgment without taking sides or appearing manipulated by circumstances. Beige provides an even playing field for conflict resolution and often bring sanity back from chaos. The Beige beauty insists on substantial quiet time—almost to the point of reclusiveness—so that she can fully enjoy the clean, uncluttered, orderly, and beatific world she creates for herself. There are many shades of beige. Each carries a base color that affects the vibrational experience in addition to beige's white base note. The cream-based warm beiges emit softer aspects of yellow, adding clarity, focus and optimism. Pink-based beiges will embody additional love vibrations. Green notes create a very harmonious and social layer to their communication style. Brown-based or gray-based beiges will send a softer note of the tint, tone, or shade added providing an invitation to be heard. Beige personalities allow for reiteration, compromise, and decompression...defusing stress and angst. She glows and brings into focus the Divine spirituality that connects us all.

## The Divine Color of NEUTRALITY and IMPARTIALITY

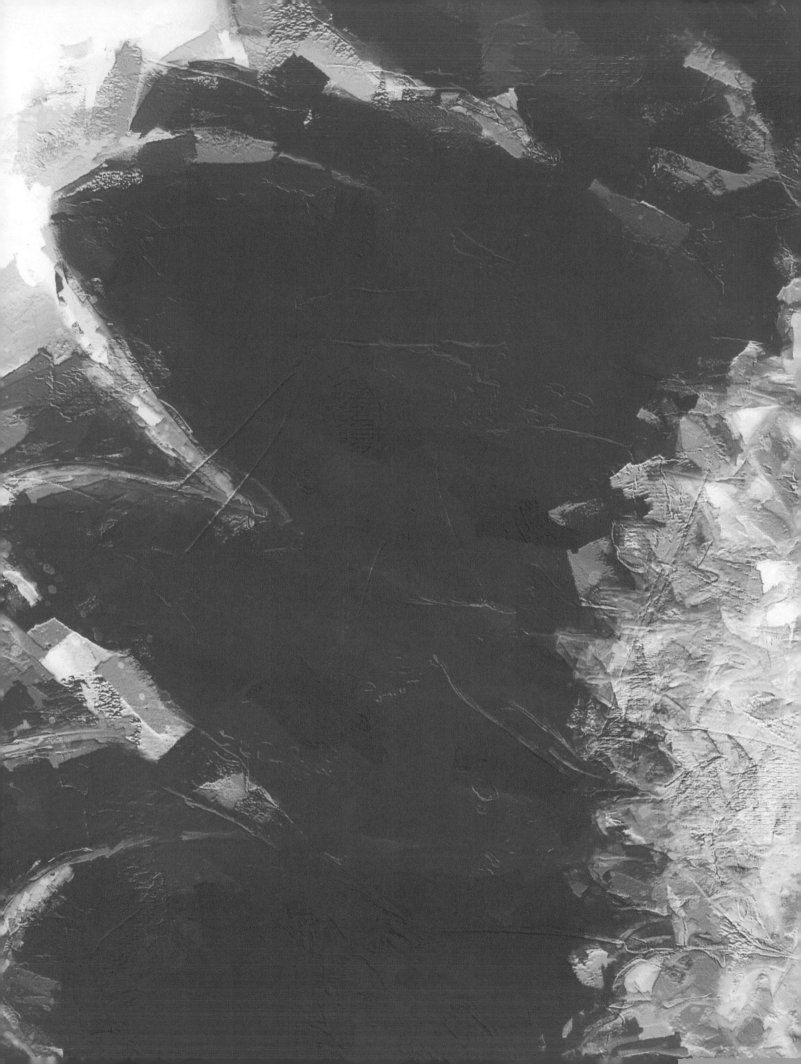

# Orange

Orange is the color of joy, happiness, enthusiasm, and fun! It is playful, appetite enhancing, and engaging. Orange souls are the happiest souls. They are life's enthusiasts. If there is a party, you will find an Orange at the center of attention, laughing and having a blast and bringing the whole room into a heightened level of play! Often a bit self-involved, but fun-loving and pure in spirit, these girls are a combination of red (they take action; let's do this now, pal) and yellow... mentally clear and as bright as the sun! Never put off 'til tomorrow the party you can enjoy today! The world needs Orange personalities to remind them to get involved, be spontaneous, and laugh out loud! Orange women live in the minute; they're very present and engaging. Their enthusiasm is infectious, their passion for enjoying every moment and activities is magnetic, and, in spite of their self-satisfying nature, they are always looking for friends to join with them to play! Oranges are social butterflies... sometimes a bit self-centered but always gregarious and generous with their time and resources.

Orange women are usually quick thinkers, focused and clear, and love action! Orange embodies the true nature of happiness. They are living and breathing natural antidepressants offering a renewed interest in life. Orange personas create fun and promote recreation and healing. They emit exuberance. Oranges are great manifesters.

## *The Divine Color of FUN, JOY, ENTHUSIASM and PLAY*

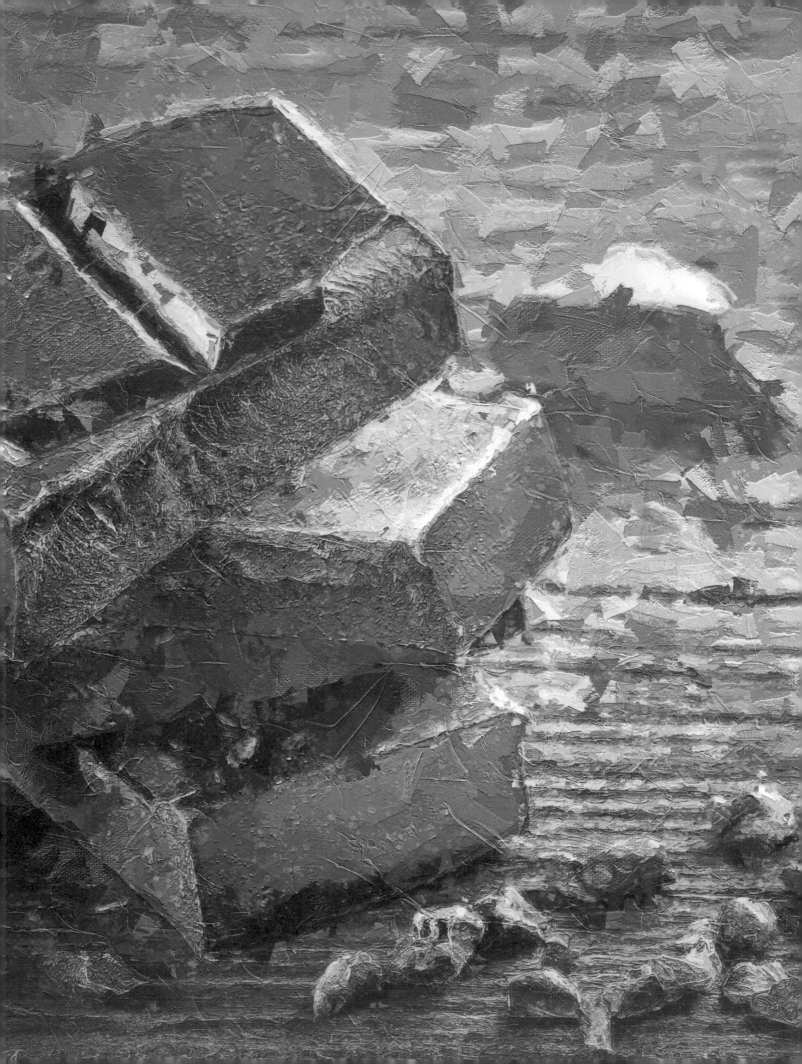

# Brown

Brown is the color of groundedness, stability, durability, practicality, and the earth. Brown provides a sense of having both feet on the ground in a very real and physical manner, providing roots to any situation and a deep sense of belonging and history. They relish in bringing people together and honoring their talents and abilities as well as their culture, personal journey, and mission. Brown personalities possess the uncanny ability to make everyone present feel secure and accepted, seen and heard. There are low-key, rarely needing to bring attention to themselves.

Some women have a certain apathy or resistance toward the color brown. I have found through my years of working in this modality that some women need grounding and are repelled by the thought of being tied down. They fully buy into the air and water and love to set sail in any direction the wind blows. They eventually discover that this attraction to living "out of their bodies" creates a certain sense of being off balance and uncentered. Hmmmm. Lots more on that for sure! Brown is necessary. If one has roots... one also has wings to fly!

Whenever you are around a Brown personality you feel safe, secure, and grounded. Their practical earthy nature is appreciated by less stable signs, and their down-to-earth, no muss/no fuss way of life and rugged temperament are admired and enjoyed. Brown personalities are rather natural in their appearance and not overly concerned by airs and attitudes. They deal firmly in reality, share the spotlight, and understand their place in the cosmos without a care of changing.

The Brown personality is content and confident. They know who they are and what they positively contribute to any situation. They tend to assemble well-balanced and high-functioning teams. Their ego is usually in check because they are deeply aware that Brown personalities provide the very ground that the world needs to walk upon! They are comfortable in their skin... and convey a sense of belonging and rootedness to others.

## The Divine Color of GROUNDEDNESS, STABILITY, SECURITY and EARTHINESS

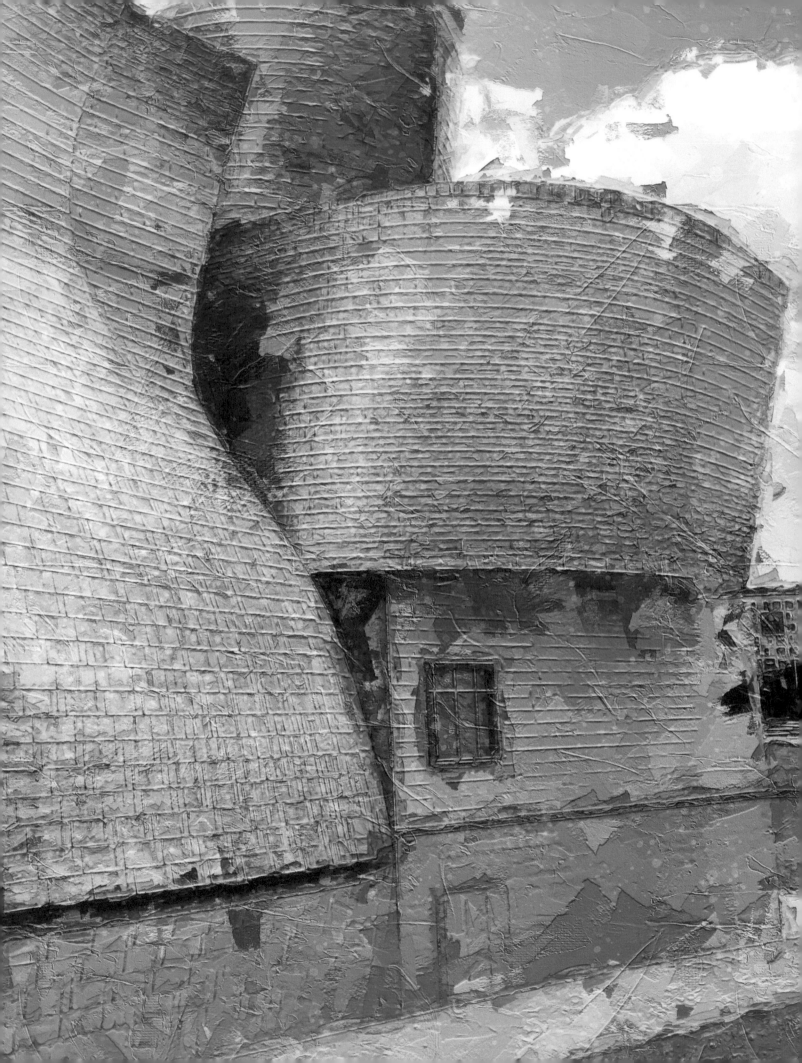

# Gray

Gray is the oddity of the Divine Color Palette. It is elusive and noncommittal, as it doesn't exist in retracted white light and therefore doesn't truly exist in the realm of divine vibrations. It is included here as an accommodation for those who are attracted to this shade and those who use it in their wardrobe, career, and lifestyle choices.

Gray is a mixture of black and white...anonymity, cloaking, and mystery along with divine understanding, enlightenment, and priority. I am sure you can see the predicament. The vibrations are juxtaposed in gray, possessing opposing emotional and vibrational messages. How can a girl be divine in nature and totally unwilling or incapable of letting her light shine? It happens every day.

Women who are attracted to gray are in a state of transition. They are in the process of choosing the highest and best for themselves and their life...thus, gray becomes a powerful tool to use for distancing herself from any emotional involvement, physical attachment, or intellectual repartee. This roadblock to the heart is intentional and should be approached with caution. Professional circumstances can be leveraged by the addition of gray into a color palette. It's a strategic color choice for an ultimate chess game.

Over the years, I have somewhat softened on my opinion of gray, discovering that, like beige, it carries energy from the top notes that are added to the black and white base notes. There is an exception to gray, here, as noted. Silver when printed provides a matte finish, which appears to be gray in many fabrications, textiles, accessories, and decorative furnishings. Silver is anything but the color of indecision. It is the gorgeous soulful color of all that is Yin in our conscious and subconsciousness.

Women who love the silver-hued, soft, sensitive gray tones that fall under the heading of silver are gifts to this world. Their energy is receptive and encouraging, warm and comforting. Silver added to any other color palette softens the energetic field, which is often an asset to the wearer. Pearl grays and soft pale pewters resonate in the silver spectrum. Please read further for more insights into the power of this beautiful hue.

## The Divine Color of NON-DECISION and NON-COMMITMENT

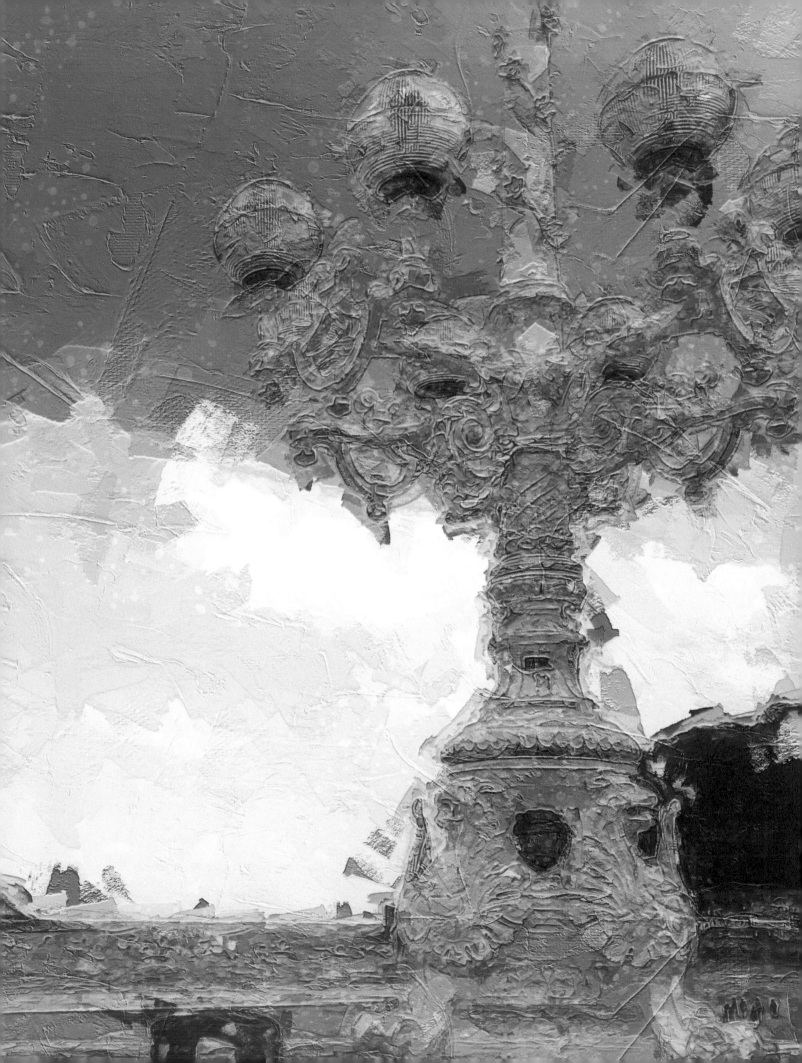

# Silver and Gold

Silver and Gold are not usually the Dominant Divine personalities but rather a sparkling layer and shimmering energy field that surrounds and emanates and deeply enhances the primary color personality. Silver and Gold Personality traits vivify what is already so abundant in a personality.

# Silver

Silver, symbolically represented by the moon, contains "the lightness of being." It speaks to femininity and a receptive nature. Silver is an all-embracing color signifying humility in character, a virtue without which the other principles cannot work effectively. Silver predicts one's unspoken nature. Silver is very much an overlay of how the world perceives our power.

Silver personalities are very nurturing and soft in their effect. They do not have to be the center of attention because they are deeply aware of the energetic field that emits from calm, serene, and life-giving forces. Along with gold, it portrays a perfect balance of joy. The Silver personality overlay offers the opportunity to receive all the feminine experiences in life—the joy of receptivity, intuition, and receiving love and gratitude.

## The Divine Color of THE YIN

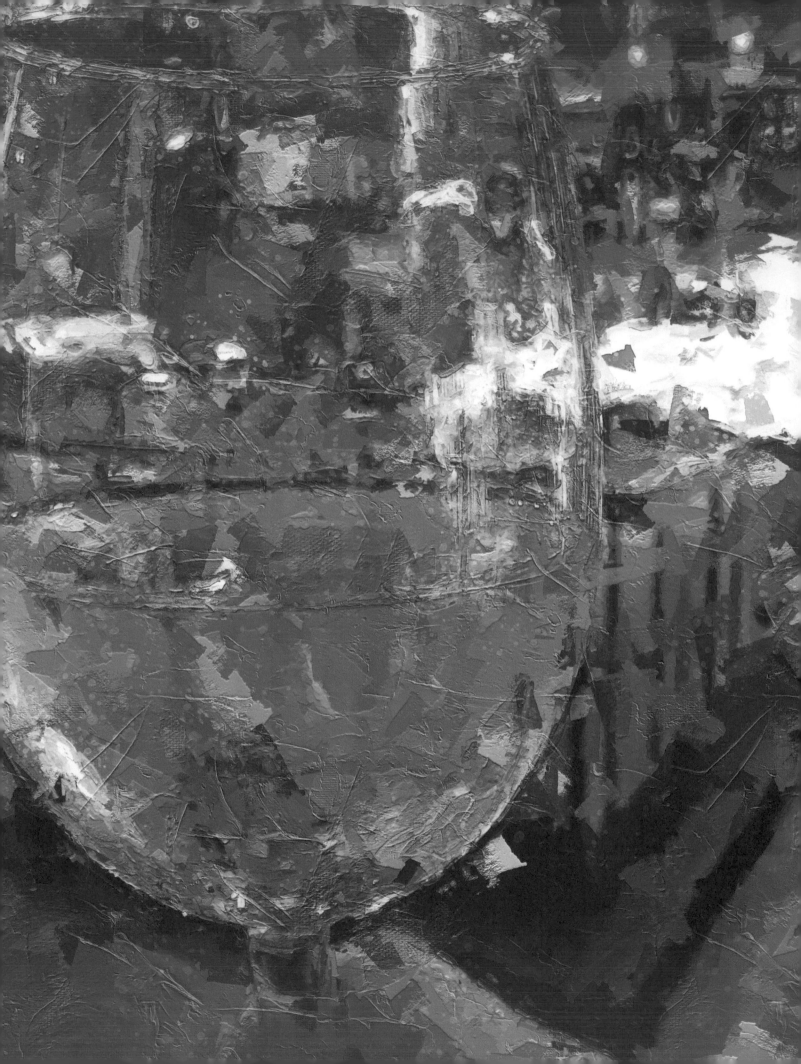

# Gold

Gold, symbolically represented by the sun, reflects all that is active and participatory in life. Power, abundance, and productivity are embraced by Gold personality overlay. Motivation and all the active principles of joy, love, and success are harnessed by this color. Gold personalities effuse Chi energy—bold and unignorable, radiant and self-assured. The Gold personality overlay emphasizes the richness and all-encompassing nature of creating. Along with Silver, it portrays the perfect union of all the colors and the sublime integration of all the vibrational Divine Color Principles. Gold reflects the possibility of manifesting life in the now moment and encourages others to embrace their masculine energy by taking action and catalyzing their Yin dreams into reality!

## The Divine Color
## of THE YANG

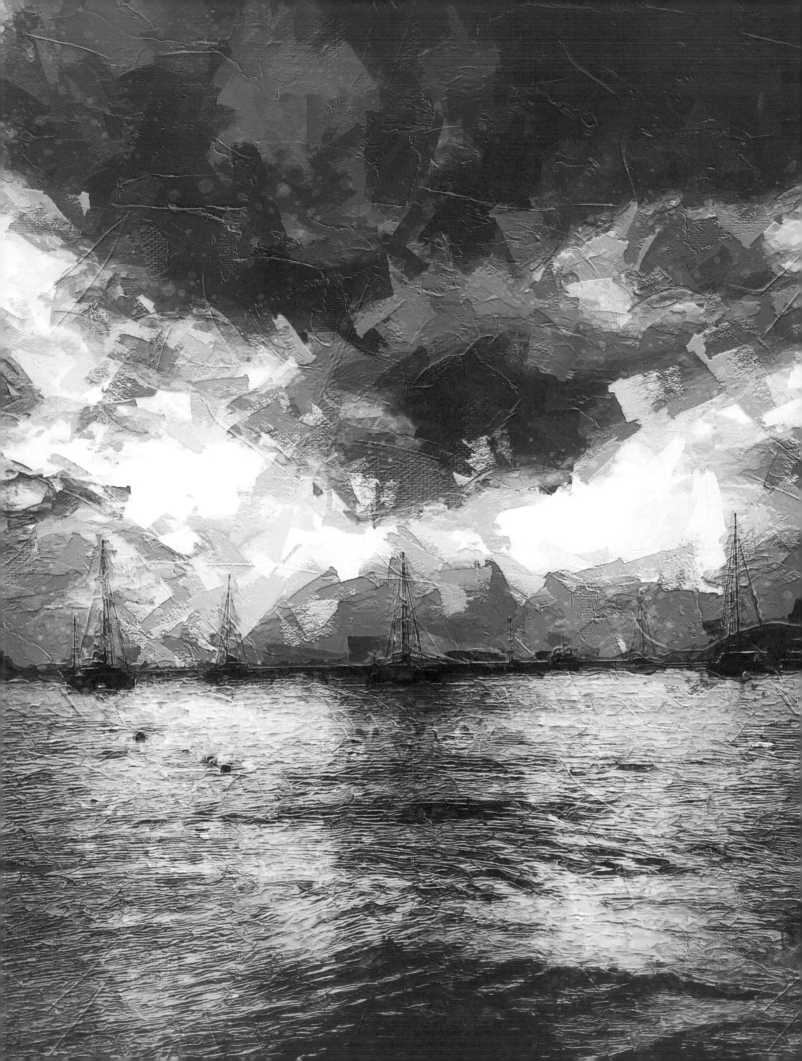

# Black

Black is not a color; rather it is the absence of color. Black is a cloaking hue, protecting the wearer from scrutiny while providing an energetic block for the garnering of any insight or invasion into the privacy or inner workings of the wearer. The color black camouflages and hides the wearer from plain sight, allowing her to go on her merry way without being noticed or seen. It gives a sense of anonymity...sometimes a little of that does a body good! This is why black is the most commonly worn color in cities like New York, where denizens like to go about their business without being noticed and intruded upon by anyone or anything. For this purpose, black is very handy and truly beneficial. If a gal does not want to attract immediate attention, black can be her best option.

The opposite is also true. Black is mysterious and impenetrable. Perhaps that is why we consider it sexy. Long live the little black dress! It allows us to be part of the group without raising too many flags, but depending on style, it also conveys a certain uniqueness, mystery, and allure, which translates as sexy and attractive. Of course, facts are facts: black does make a girl appear more slender, and for that reason it will always be alive and well in all of our closets! It travels well. It hides a multitude of sins. It is seasonless and goes with every other shade of color.... Raise your hand if you agree. Black has its place... and I am raising a glass in homage to its magical powers!

## The Divine Color of PROTECTION, ANONYMITY and MYSTERY

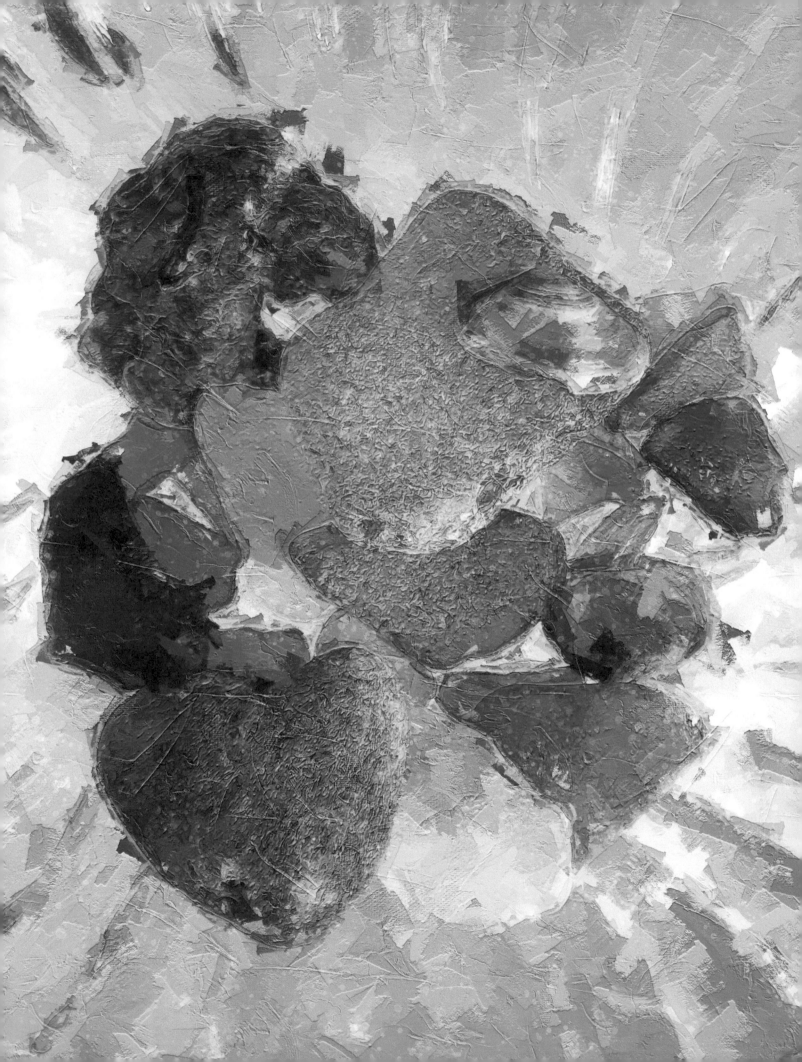

# Let's Recap

There is a Divine Color within in each of us that emanates from deep within our soul and vibrates at a certain frequency, attracting certain people and experiences and repelling others. Each of us manifests our life in accordance with our soul colors when we discover the rainbow of opportunity that lies within our grasp. Once we embrace and accept the challenge of creating our perfect prismatic vibration by integrating all the colors of the spectrum, each vibrating in perfect harmony with our being, we will function at our highest, happiest and most fulfilling frequency. We will attract love, joy, success, and abundance into our lives.

The color lessons included above give you the first hints in understanding the colors within your soul and the same guidelines as to what colors work best for your personal brand and success in the world. What happens if the colors our audience needs to see and the colors we need to wear to be our best and most vibrant self, clash? Do we sacrifice our sense of well-being and risk failure by ignoring our own needs to satisfy our audience? NOT AT ALL!!!! We know that in order to be our best personally and publicly we must be authentic and transparent and live at our highest vibration, emanating our most dynamic presence. So how do we achieve color harmony? By understanding the world of color and incorporating both our personal and professional best colors into our zeitgeist, we can achieve maximum results before we even say a word!! That is the power of color!

Have you figured out who you might be in the rainbow spectrum of divine colors? Do you have a strong attraction to a certain hue? Hopefully, you have gained insight into what each of the colors symbolize and convey to the observer and support for the wearer. This is a huge topic and deserves its very own book...

For now, I wanted to introduce you to your palette preferences and share how powerful wearing, seeing, touching, eating and experiencing color is in your life. I want you to feel empowered by having the choice to wear a color that expresses to the world who you are and what you want to accomplish personally and professionally. Equipped with this knowledge, you can truly influence and direct another person's thoughts and actions to achieve your ultimate goals! Manipulation... I would never say such things... Ultimate persuasion? Absolutely.... *A woman has to have as many tricks up her sleeve as possible.*

# CHAPTER 26

*The Gentle Art of Color Persuasion*

Here is my little list on the art of nonverbal communication through color. It will come in handy next time you are selecting an outfit for an important calendar date.

## Mary's Curated Art of Color Persuasion

Being empowered and equipped for a personal or professional meeting is as simple as: knowing your stuff, bringing your "A" game, and wearing the right outfit in the perfect shade of persuasion!

*What color to wear when you want someone to:*

Trust you: BLUE

Feel good about themselves: PINK

Feel alert and focused on what you're saying: YELLOW

Have optimal communication: TURQUOISE

Act NOW: RED

Feel peaceful: GREEN

Have fun: ORANGE

Feel healthy and vital: GREEN

Feel creative: PURPLE

Know that you are powerful: RED, BRIGHT PINK, WHITE, ELECTRIC BLUE

Be intimidated and know that you are serious: BLACK

Feel loved: PINK

Know that you feel confident and self-assured: WHITE

Know that you are a team player: BLUE

Know that you are loyal: BLUE

Feel forgiveness: PURPLE

Join in on a new adventure: ORANGE

Feel mentally inspired: BLUE

Feel understood, heard, and valued: DUSTY SHADES OF BLUE, PINK, LAVENDER

Feel sexy and alluring: RED

Feel physically invigorated and fully alert: RED

Feel a sense of openness, acceptance, no partiality, or judgment: BEIGE

Feel comfortable and easygoing: GREEN

Feel rugged and capable: BROWN

Feel positive: YELLOW

Feel totally empowered in an active way: GOLD

Feel totally empowered in a passive, reflective way: SILVER

Know that you are practical, stable, and grounded: BROWN

*Being empowered and equipped for a personal or professional meeting is as simple as: knowing your stuff, bringing your "A" game, and wearing the right outfit in the perfect shade of persuasion!*

Feel connected to the earth: BROWN

Feel safe: BLUE and PINK

Take risks: RED

Feel spiritually inspired: PURPLE

Feel calm and meditative: PURPLE, INDIGO, MAGENTA

Feel refreshed and energized: TURQUOISE

Know that you are the "real deal": BLUE, PEACH

Feel hungry: ORANGE, RED

Attract volunteers and "do-gooders": GREEN

Feel orderly: YELLOW, BEIGE

Feel solitude: WHITE

Feel hopeful: YELLOW

Feel in touch with the Divine: WHITE

Remember that these are general recommendations and that each particular situation will call for adjustments, tonal balance, and special considerations, especially when combining colors for your greatest success!

Here are 18 Golden Rules of Choosing The Best Colors for Your Wardrobe. They are steadfast, true and important to consider when purchasing your clothing and accessories for your personal and professional life. Social media gives a microphone and stage to anyone who has the desire to share their passion and promise to the world. Some of these rules have direct impact on the power of non-verbal communication in media.

1.  The brighter the color, the more intense the impact and emotion connected to the color.

2.  "Listener" colors have gray added. They are subtler and less controlling and encourage open communication. These colors should be worn when a compassionate understanding and active listening are needed to enhance healing on any level.

3.  "Speaker" colors are pure hues or have black/gray added. They should be worn when the communicator is sharing significant information and is the center of attention for a designated period of time.

4.  The more white a color has in it, the softer the effect.

5.  Red and white enlarge and expand in media, photography, video and TV, as do most brights.

6.  Black and dark colors diminish and reduce.

7.  The neutral colors used for negative space are as important as the colors chosen for positive space.

8.  Your favorite color may not be the best color choice for your being or brand.

9.  Sometimes a color combination is more powerful and effective than the use of a single color.

10. Three colors are optimal for a wardrobe and a personal brand strategy.

11. When in doubt, go with solids, not prints. Solids are always preferable to prints on camera, in photos and on TV.

*Social media gives a microphone and stage to anyone who has the desire to share their passion and promise with the world.*

12. Colors can exhaust the viewer if the exposure is too long or big. Be careful with the use of red, orange, and yellow.

13. Getting someone's attention and keeping their attention often requires a palette change.

14. The best greens are always blue green—not yellow green like mustard. Think of nature. The purer the hue, the clearer the message.

15. The best on-camera colors are blue, green, turquoise, and yellow. Orange and red are now very wearable thanks to HD cameras as well as most any color on the spectrum.

16. Your best white should enhance the whiteness of your teeth and naturally up-light your skin undertone. Most people's best white is not pure white. it is a shade off—either creamy or taupe depending upon the undertone color of your skin pigment.

17. If you are exceptionally tall, you can use color blocking to lessen your visual image by wearing contrasting colors separating your top and bottom half. Similarly, you can achieve a taller visual image by wearing a monochromatic look from head to toe. Also, you can expand or shrink your width by using color blocking and focusing color down the center or down the outline of your frame and contrasting that color with a darker neutral. These optical illusions are enhanced by your color choices. Everyone can take full advantage of utilizing color to balance their image.

18. Different nations have different color biases, interpretations, and usages. If you are branding globally, it is important to consider the cultural overlays of your color choices before fully implementing them into your brand formula. I am using the color overlays for the United States in these exercises and suggestions. Culturally, social mores have an extremely significant effect on public opinion. Consider these before traveling to speak outside the US, and adapt your wardrobe and marketing piece to reflect and respect your host country's natural biases.

These are guidelines for you to apply when considering color choices for both your professional and personal life. There are exceptions to every single rule—even these that I created with your success in mind. A word to the wise...

## Love in the Glossy Sheets

When I first created this modality, I was asked to be a guest on The Montel Williams Show. It was such a blast! We did two segments. Montel went into the audience and asked me to interpret audience members' outfits du jour and what it conveyed about their authentic nature! It was so "spot on" and hilarious that I felt like the Color Psychic. At that moment I realized that this color concept was so much bigger than life! It really works!

In areas of the heart, and in the days of light-speed dating and virtual matchmaking, it is more important than ever to make sure that how you represent yourself projects who you really are in person. Color and style are essential factors in attracting your perfect potential partner.

I am not suggesting that you query your dates about their favorite colors and try to analyze their conscious and subconscious minds on your initial meeting. This will lead to total failure, I promise you. Not only will they think you are crazy, you most probably will be wrong about your conclusions. Stick to the basics.... Let's stick with your wardrobe choices and how they affect whom you meet.

Brown is a bit BOOOOOOORRRING for a first date.... Grounded and stable is not what they have on their mind...

Pink is for romance and true love.

Red is for passion in action and perhaps a little foray. It can also be translated as PURE power and control, so if you like to run the show and be on top, this could work both ways.

Purple can be a bit intimidating, unless of course the person you are questioning loves purple too!

Blue is for true blue. Marriage material. Miss Suzy Sensible, at your service.

Orange is let's have pure fun—insta happy and selfie time!

*What lifestyle and personality*
*are you communicating?*
*Let's dress for the kind of partner who*
*will provide the relationship we seek.*

Green is for altruists. If you want to date a humanitarian or a do-gooder, wearing green will attract all kinds of volunteers and devotees in the balancing act of life.

Black is very alluring. What they don't know is always more interesting than what they do know...

The big consideration is this: What kind of partner are you looking for? What qualities do you admire? What lifestyle and personality arc you communicating? So many women, including myself, are caught wearing things that attract the wrong type of person and then we act all shocked and surprised when we get the response we are dressed to elicit! If you can't handle the heat, girls, get out of the fire. Dressing too provocatively can attract lots of opportunities. Let's dress for the kind of partner who will provide the relationship we seek.

Now that you have a clear stream of consciousness about your authentic self, make sure that your online presence and real-time wardrobe is in alignment with your hopes and dreams and values. So many women post photos that have nothing to do with who they truly are and then wonder why things go south so soon. Be yourself. If you show up trying to be anything but your authentic self, the results will be dismal. There is someone out there for you! Until that time comes and even if it never comes... know that the only relationship that really matters is the one that you have with yourself. Once we love ourselves, the rest falls into place.

Undeniably You! was written for you to strip away all the judgments, misunderstandings, fashion disasters, makeup, and goo. Undeniably You! offers the opportunity, know-how, and support to create your authentic being and live the life of your dreams. If you are looking for a keeper, better start dressing like one.

Line
Shape
Color
Texture
Form
Value
and
Space

# CHAPTER 27

## How Line, Color and Shape Can Be Your Best Fashion Influencers

My passion for fashion has a lot to do with my passion for art. I firmly believe that a woman can and should own art, touch art, eat art, hear art, wear art, and actually BE art. The key to creating an unforgettable persona and an exquisite image is to create a masterpiece from the inside out that tells your story effortlessly and effusively.

Who are your favorite artists and why are you attracted to their art? Your answers reveal a lot about yourself. You identify with art that resonates with your soul. Can you imagine how powerful your presence will be once you consider yourself a visual masterpiece? Let's talk about art to wear, the art of dressing, and the culling and curating of your unique masterpiece, your style DNA.

Each of the 7 elements of art—Line, Shape, Color, Texture, Form, Value, and Space—offers essential elements in creating a masterpiece. These elements also exist in fashion design. Once you have a working knowledge of this vocabulary and concept, it will be easy breezy to use this book to help chart your course to success. Let's take them, one by one, and describe why they are an essential part of looking fabulous and feeling great.

Mathematics and fashion go hand in hand. Let's discuss the way simple geometry and shapes, pattern, line, and form can achieve your best silhouette depending on your authentic personal style formula. Your archetype, style persona, body type, skin coloring, and divine color vibration all factor in to determine the creation of your being as art, as well as the overall look that you are hoping to achieve through your wardrobe.

*Vertical lines elongate.*
*Horizontal lines add width.*
*Diagonal lines create curves.*

## Line

A line takes the viewer's eye for a walk. Simply put, that is exactly what lines in fashion catalyze... they direct our vision to a completion point. Our job is to predetermine what their eyes are moving toward and exactly what they will see at the end of their walk.

In fashion, a line refers to an elongated band that connects two or more points. Line in fashion can be created by the structure or embellishment features of a garment. Structural lines are created by the cut of the garment. Lines have direction (vertical, horizontal, diagonal, curvy, jagged) and weight (thick, thin). Lines can create an illusion. One's figure can appear taller and slimmer or broader and even curvier.

The use of geometry in fashion can trick the eye into focusing on specific body parts and enlarge, diminish, lengthen, and shorten the appearance of a figure's proportions drastically. Models have used this technique for decades, drawing the viewer's eye to what we want them to see and camouflaging those aspects of ourselves that are out of balance or less attractive. Magicians call it sleight of hand; artists refer to it as trompe-l'oeil. All in all, it is the fine art of distraction and seduction. Within a garment's flirt with reality, all of our bodies seem divine.

For example, vertical unbroken lines that span from shoulder to hemline—evenly spaced and proportionate to the figure size—will convey the notion that a person is taller and slimmer. Horizontal lines will expand whatever area of the body that they are covering. A woman with larger hips and a smaller bust might wear a horizontal striped top with a width of stripe that is proportional to her frame. This perfect geometry will balance an imbalanced natural figure. It will "expand" the shoulder and bust area by drawing the viewer's eye to it in a left to right motion. And it will diminish the viewer's attention paid to the hip by making it "recede."

The human eye wants to resolve everything it sees. The human eye seeks to achieve balance. Once we learn how to use lines and patterns to assist the viewer's eye in achieving visual symmetry, we convey a sense of harmony in our figure.

Using line and form is a wonderful game of "smoke and mirrors." We diminish the areas of our figure that are not perfect by drawing attention away from them and drawing attention to the figure facets that are lovelier. We focus on our best and camouflage the rest.

A woman with an ample bust and/or broad shoulders and narrow hips can easily create balance by wearing a solid-colored top and matching it with striped or patterned pants or skirt. A woman can also "narrow" the shoulders by interrupting the visual field with a colored shirt, V-neck or opened jacket, or sweater worn over a shell in a contrasting color. The vertical line created by showing a bit of décolleté narrows the viewer's visual plane. An over sweater or jacket gives the illusion that the space underneath is narrower than it truly measures. The vertical lines of the jacket or sweater can break up the broadness of the shoulder or the bustline. The eye automatically brings the shoulder visually closer to balance the frame.

Straight vertical lines tend to work best on figures that are more straight than curvy. The curvier the figure, the more careful one must be with vertical fields. Curvy or diagonal lines can work beautifully on a curvy shape.

Horizontal lines work ever so well on straighter figures but have their place in the sun with curvy girls as long as the width of the line is proportionate to the body's overall size and height. Broad, big lines on a diminutive figure make us look like we borrowed someone else's clothes. Skinny lines with a constant repeat on a large frame will make someone look like a circus tent and cause the viewer to feel seasick. The larger the frame, the larger the line. The smaller the frame, the smaller the line. The more space between the lines, the more control you have over diminishing the overall look.

Vertical lines elongate. Horizontal lines add width. Diagonal lines create curves. The overall line of a dress describes how a garment is designed. Lines as print also have a huge visual effect.

## Shape and Form

To simplify our immediate conversation, I am collapsing shape and form into one definition. The shape is the outward appearance of a garment, its form or silhouette observed as an overall outline. The shape is created by the cut and construction of a garment. Form expresses the external appearance of a clearly defined area, as distinguished by cut, color, or fabric.

There are dozens of classic shapes in fashion that assist us in describing the overall appearance of a garment. In dresses, these silhouettes include A-line, empire, sheath, princess, shift, wrap, bodycon, halter, peplum, baby doll, mermaid, shirt waist, ball gown, trapeze, asymmetrical, and slip. There are so many more terms for every type of garment. This is just a start to illustrate the language of clothing. Every type of garment falls into a silhouette. Necklines, pants, sweaters, blouses use descriptive terms for easy reference.

I refer to these shapes to assist your understanding of perfect choices for your perfect silhouette. Every design house creates specific silhouettes, which makes their brand and fit memorable and unique.

Each body type looks best in specific shapes and forms, accenting the best features. Once you recognize and understand which silhouettes work best for your body and person, shopping becomes a breeze and you will have the confidence in your purchasing power.

And while we are on the topic of shape, great shapewear can transform your life. Everyone needs a little "pick me up," "push me in," or "smooth me over" power assist when creating your best looks. Invest in top quality foundations, girls. Buy a gold standard bra that lifts and supports your breasts. It will instantly take off ten years and ten pounds along with locating your long-lost waistline! If the undergarment isn't right, the outfit will never look right on you. Your carriage and esteem will soar once you see yourself dressed and supported by the right bra and panties.

## Color and Value

Color can be defined as the quality of a substance with respect to the light reflected by the object, usually determined visually by measurement of hue, saturation, and brightness of the reflected light; saturation or chroma. In fashion, as in life, color is the number one reason people are attracted to or repelled by something. Color, as we have discussed, carries a vibrational charge that nonverbally informs the viewer and the wearer of spiritual and emotional vibrational charges.

In fashion, color has a multitude of interpretations and uses. For the purpose of our discussion, we will only consider a few main themes surrounding color use and placement so that we can utilize colors to attain the overall look that we desire for our wardrobe. Color has many components. The basic terms are Hue, Value, Tint, Tone and Shade and Saturation. We explored this in the Seasonal Chapter. Now let's discuss how color affects the overall appearance of our figure when placed in particular areas and order.

Let's discuss two powerful and effective ways to utilize color to bring out the best in you: Color Blocking and Monochromatic Dressing. Color blocking, the use of juxtaposing complementary colors, can be used to exaggerate or diminish a body part. Reds, yellows, and oranges visually expand an area. Blues, greens, and purples diminish an area. White brings an image forward, enlarging it. Black causes a feature to visually recede, reducing its appearance.

When used properly, along with proportion and line, colors can become a girl's best friend. A color will bring the viewer's eye to accentuate your positives and reduce the visual space of the negatives. It can also broaden or narrow the entire field. Place the boldest, largest blocks of color on the body parts you would like to celebrate. Use the quieter, smaller blocks to quietly tone down the areas you would like to go unnoticed.

## *Let's explore my ready rules to color-block your body like a pro.*

**Monochromatic Dressing** uses one color and/or shades of the same color to achieve an overall cohesive look that can lengthen, slenderize, and expand based upon line choice. Select the lighter shades for areas that should be accented and place the darker shades in areas that need to recede. Honing your knowledge of line and proper color placement will give you the most attractive overall visual statement.

**Color Blocking** allows you to use colors that are separated but not equal. Mix garments by using two to four colors that either complement or contrast, tricking the eye into believing that certain features are larger and others smaller. Several designers are using color blocking with panache, deliberately creating the perfect visual effect for your fashion pleasure. Piet Mondrian, a Dutch painter, explored the use of the opposite colors on the color wheel and pairing them to make interesting combinations. In fashion history, Yves Saint Laurent was the first to debut the use of color blocking when he emulated Mondrian's painting as a dress in his 1946 fall winter show.

**Color Field Painting**, as it was once known, is using significant areas of a single color juxtaposed to another color to bring about a visual and emotional event or response, harnessing the power of color, unrestricted by line or form, to create an expression. Mark Rothko, one of the most well-known abstract expressionists in the '40s and '50s, used color blocking in his work to act as a catalyst for generating pure emotion from his viewers. Later, in the '60s and '70s, color blocking was used as an expression of emotion and experimentation as this generation emerged with a passion for individuality,

*The texture stimulates*
*two different senses: sight and touch.*
*Texture also describes*
*the surface appearance of fabric.*
*Texture is the one element*
*you can see and feel.*
*Texture is found in the thickness*
*and appearance of the fabric*
*and any embellishments.*

modernity, and freedom, from Peter Max to Warhol and so many other contemporary designers. Today, color blocking and monochromatic fashion is the rage. Gorgeous collections are found everywhere and at every price point.

## Texture

Texture in painting refers to the look and feel of the canvas. It is based on the paint, and its application, or the addition of materials such as ribbon, metal, wood, lace, leather, and sand. The concept of "painterliness" also has bearing on texture. The texture stimulates two different senses: sight and touch. Texture also describes the surface appearance of fabric. Texture is the one element you can see and feel. Texture is found in the thickness and appearance of the fabric and any embellishments.

Words that describe texture are: loopy, fuzzy, furry, soft, shiny, dull, bulky, rough, crisp, smooth, sheer, etc. Certain bulky textures, such as brocade and boucle, add volume to a figure. Smoother textures, such as silk, knits, gabardines, and jersey with the addition of spandex, minimize a figure's volume. Texture is a spectacular way to harness emotion and express personal style in your wardrobe. Perhaps that is why textures of all fabrications and descriptions flood the runways.

## Space

Filled space and empty space are referred to a positive space and negative space. Clothing designers use the negative and positive space associated with shapes to create a surface design or pattern. The concept of space goes hand in hand with the concepts of color placement, noted above in our discussion of monochroma, and color blocking. Space can also be used to enlarge or diminish a specific area. Oftentimes, negative space colors are considered to be the neutral garment color, which plays against a featured accent color. In times past, black, navy, gray, white, taupe, and beige were most often considered as neutrals. Today, any color can be used as the main theme or "neutral" dominant color story. Contrasting accent colors are then selected to "pop" or accentuate a design feature. The choice of the negative space color will determine whether that area of the body will visually recede, diminish or expand, come forward.

Once upon a time, fashion dictated strict rules for seasonal attire. These rules are long gone. There are no steadfast rules for when or how to use color in your wardrobe. Wardrobe Capsule Dressing utilizes space by dictating a neutral or core color for creating multiple "looks" or outfits that go together seamlessly. The only rule that I impose is that whatever colors we choose to wear should make us look our best.

That's a wrap, ladies, on the basic construction tools we use to create your image as art. I would suggest you take a stroll to a nearby gallery or museum and discover which artists and paintings tug at your heartstrings and set your soul on fire. Experience the art without judgment or thought and simply allow the art to speak to you. Make a note of the pieces that are aligned with your spiritual nature. Why are you attracted to them and how do they make you feel? Is it the line that attracts your eye? Is it the use of color, shape, or texture? What about the artworks catalyze an emotional response? Are those feelings something that you would like to portray in your visual grammar? What do they say about you?

Once you start understanding the inner nature of your image as art and add that language to your personal style formula,  you will start to create your truly authentic you! Art informs your self-awareness and can influence your personal style.

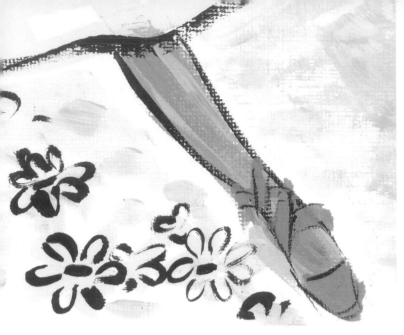
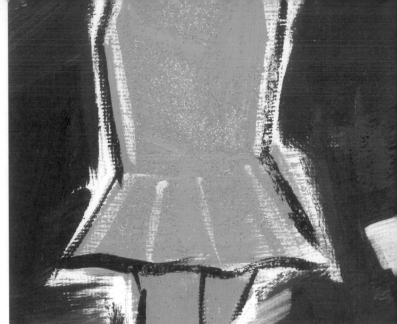
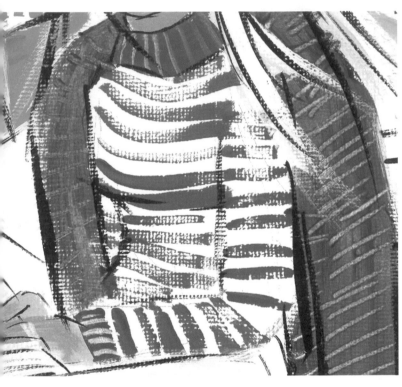
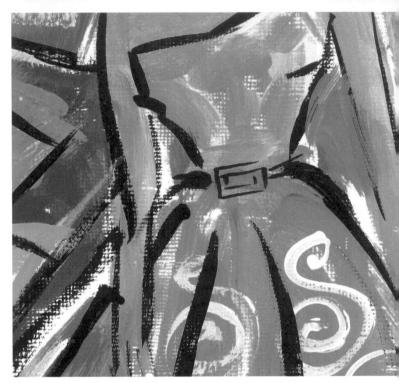
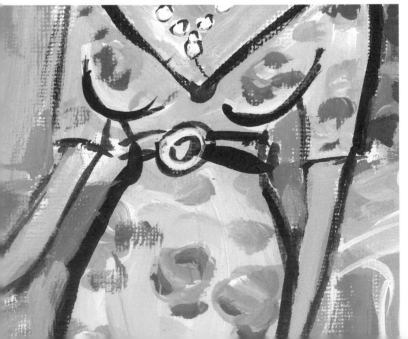
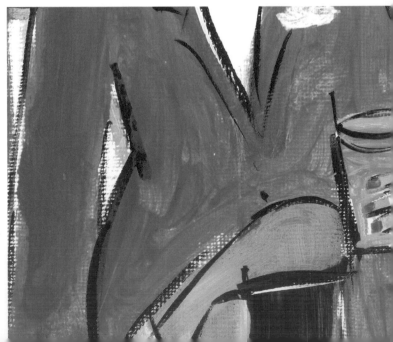

# CHAPTER 28
## Wardrobe Capsule Dressing

It's no secret, and it's making a huge comeback. Wardrobe Capsule Dressing will save you time, money, stress, your dignity, and, perhaps, your job. It's easy, breezy, and cost efficient. Today many designers ascribe to this sensible and evergreen philosophy of becoming well-heeled in one easy shopping excursion.

Capsule Dressing is the only way to leave the house or hotel in the early morning and return late at night without ever feeling inappropriately attired, miss-appointed, or faded. Your transitions from morning to evening and business to social hours can be as effortless as a few things in a tote bag. You will always look fabulous and you will never look outdated or outmaneuvered by your closet.

How? It's the best kept secret in the business and now the formula is yours. Welcome to the club! We travel with a carry-on and carry on as we pretty please wherever and whenever we like. Here is the key: 20 pieces that are totally interchangeable and season-less (at least three seasons of wearability) and classic in style, perfectly fitting and packable. This concept works for every archetype and style persona. As a matter of fact, it is the way to put your newly learned knowledge to the test. Can you create a 20-piece wardrobe as your authentic self, in your season, for your body type and with your divine colors? Can you shop on budget and without stress?

Let's get started on creating how you can look gorgeous and feel great. Yes, this system is an investment, but it will never let you down. These pieces will not replace your gym clothes and bathrobe, but they will replace all those clothes that you bought and never wear because they just don't seem to "go with anything."

*Here is the key:*
*20 pieces that are totally*
*interchangeable and seasonless*
*and classic in style,*
*perfectly fitting and packable.*

## Budget

Once you have defined your Archetype, Style Persona, Body Type, Season, and Divine Color Palette, it is time to find the resources for creating your wardrobe capsule. Set a realistic budget for your investment. Quality counts here. These pieces should last you at least three to five years depending upon how you care for them and how much you wear each piece. Some women are harder on their clothes than others. Take this into consideration.

## Color

The first choice in creating your ultimate wardrobe capsule collection is color.

1. Select your best neutral based upon the formula you have created. Black, beige, navy, brown, or matte silver are the most flexible and popular. Occasionally denim can be a primary color depending upon your style persona, lifestyle, and wardrobe needs. Your best neutral can really be any color that you adore, looks awesome, and emits the frequency that supports your essence. Red, green, turquoise, pink, yellow, orange... they are all potential neutrals. The choice is yours. Making sure that the shades are an exact match is the most important consideration when selecting an active color to be your neutral.

2. Select your best white depending upon your coloring and teeth color. Some seasons look best in pure white. Other people look best in a cream. Still others do best in a gray white or pale taupe white.

3. Select an accent or trend color. This color can change from season to season. It will keep your wardrobe fresh and updated without you needing to rebuy an entirely new wardrobe every other season.

## Fabric

I am a big fan of natural fabrics with a touch of microfiber added for comfort, fit, and packing. The base can be cotton, wool, silk, cashmere, or a totally synthetic blend. Knits, jerseys, gabardines, and microfibers all work well. The most important factor to consider is your internal and external climate. I am a big layering fan. Even though my hot flashes finally stopped, I am freezing in the air conditioning and usually hot outside.

## Proportion and Line

Make sure the clothes you purchase fit the overall line, size, and shape of your body. Refer back to Body Type to clarify the proportions that work best for your figure.

## Design Houses

Each design house has a customer avatar in mind when creating a collection. Every designer has a specific niche, figure, budget, look, and lifestyle. Editorial campaigns and fashion shows introduce their season's offerings on runway models who are not the average woman. The actual ready-to-wear collections that are delivered to stores follow the form of a specific body type and are made using "fit models" that resemble the customers who will buy the garments. Once you discover the clothing lines who design for your body type and lifestyle, shopping becomes so much easier and your success rate will soar.

Shopping within a singular line will also ensure that the fabrics, textures, colors, lines, and proportions work together to convey a pulled-together and fully coordinated look. Many designers understand the needs and desires of loyal customers and intentionally create collections that follow the rules for Wardrobe Capsule Dressing. Core color palettes remain the same from season to season, so that their buyers can maintain basic pieces and amplify their look each season with confidence and ease.

Here is the formula for creating a wardrobe capsule utilizing 20 pieces that will actually interchangeably produce up to 40 different looks and variations for all occasions and seasons. It is perfect for women who have no time to think about what they are going to put on in the morning. It is a "press play" moment and provides a no-stress start to the day! This concept also works divinely for women who travel frequently for work or pleasure or anyone whose tastes exceed their closet restrictions. Have fun. Let's get dressed the way you want to be addressed.

*Yes, this system is an investment,*
*but it will never let you down.*

## The 20 Essential Pieces

These are the key ingredients for creating your perfect "go-to" wardrobe. I suggest that you select a single designer and a specific time and date to create your capsule. Start with their "basics" or "essentials" line and grow your collection from that vantage point. Certain lines make it very easy to accomplish this exercise across all sizes and personas.

**1 Jacket**
**2 Sweaters (one can be part of a set)**
**1 Wrap**
**2 Skirts**
**2 Pants (one can be leggings)**
**2 Dresses**
**4 tops (one can be part of a sweater set)**
**3 pairs of shoes—high heels, flats and sandals, or boots**
**1 purse with a detachable smaller one inside**
**1 outerwear piece**
**1 statement accessory piece set and/or watch**

This is the very basic concept. The more pieces added to the core group, the greater the number of variations for a truly full and varied wardrobe.

*This is the formula
for creating a wardrobe capsule
utilizing 20 pieces that will actually
interchangeably produce up to
40 different looks and variations
for all occasions and seasons...
It is a "press play" moment
and provides a no-stress
start to the day!*

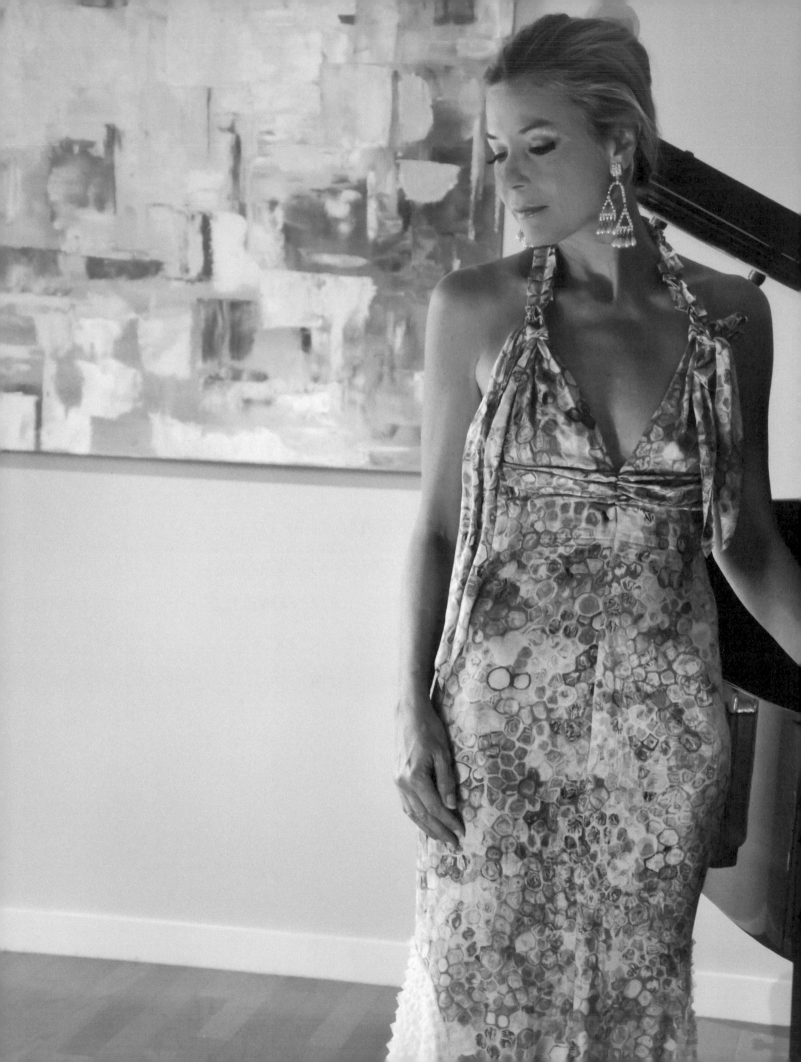

# CHAPTER 29
## The Finale

You are standing front and center, gazing at the altar of infinite potentials, basking in the glow of sacred prayer.

Longing for the answers to come to you quickly, totally unaware that they have always been there all along.

You now acknowledge that the wisdom you sought was merely shrouded by the noise of influences and critiques that shadowed and triggered your insecurities.

Lights on.

Breathe in.

Stand tall.

Just before the music starts, there you are, victorious in your persona, flawless in your fashion, celebrating your unique voice and presence.

You are poised to prance. In the spotlight, You are doing what you do best. Being undeniably you!

Deep within you radiates a Divine awareness that speaks softly as you fall asleep and is even amplified now that you are fully awake.

This is your moment.
This is your grand entrance.
This is your runway.
You are fully self-aware.
Your body, mind, and spirit are integrated.
Your inner and outer reality are in synchronicity.

You are embracing your entire being and when you see yourself in the mirror reflection, you are joyful and present and a bit amazed experiencing the fullness of your being.

No comparisons, no complaints, no critiques.
You are making your entrance.
You are communicating your intentions.
You are expecting a standing ovation.
You are prepared for your pass.
Every day is a new show and you are the VIP.
See it. Sense it. Strut it.

You Have Created Your Formula for Being Undeniably You:

# *Archetype + Style Persona + Frame + Seasonal Tonality + Divine Colors = Your Authentic Self*

Bravo! I am so proud of you!

Celebrate yourself every day.
Stay in an expression of gratitude and abundance.
Accept the notion that you are worthy of a limitless life.
Fall in love with yourself every minute.
Live with intention.
Dress for every occasion.
Recognize every success.
Experience is your teacher.
Live vividly every moment.
Choose the highest and best.

Your audience is waiting for you! And for those who can't see you and will never know your fabulousness, I only have one thing to say, "FIDO! Forget It and them and Dance On!"

*Take a bow. You are undeniably, fabulously, finally YOU!*

# BIO
## Mary Giuseffi

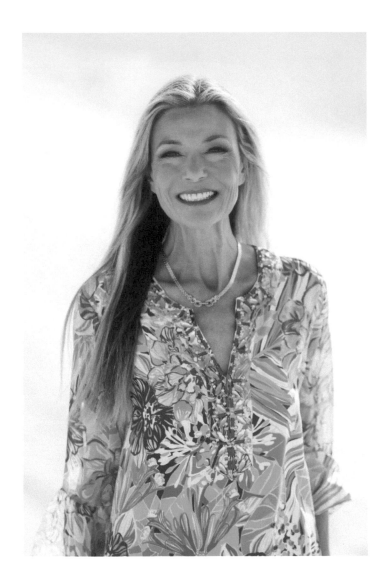

Mary Giuseffi is a Personal Brand Expert, two-time Amazon #1 Best Selling Author, Speaker, Fashion and Color Authority and Award-Winning Humanitarian and Advocate for Women and Children. She is an internationally recognized guest on many stages and TV shows, most recently The Today Show, sharing her expertise on Personal Branding and Relationships. She appears across the broadcast platforms and speaks nation-wide on Personal Branding and Marketing, Fashion and Style, Color, Self-Empowerment, and Women's inspiration

A former Ford Model and Producer, Mary's extensive experience in fashion and knowledge of beauty, on camera expertise and style sensibilities makes her a highly sought-after consultant, confidante, and coach. She is the Coach's Coach. Her consulting business spans the globe having recently created exclusive personal brands and marketing strategies for several #1 Best Selling Authors, Experts, Entrepreneurs and Reality TV Stars.

Having been on all sides of the camera for decades, she is dedicated to utilizing her talents to capture, articulate and catalyze her client's gifts and talents by bringing them to the world in a unique, authentic and powerful way. She purposefully and profoundly co-creates their Divine Purpose by creating "Sound Bites and Site Bites" to super charge their lives and careers, media presence and effectiveness as authentic dynamic personas and experts in their field.

Mary has produced and directed extraordinary fashion show productions and performance art spectacles. She served as Director of Saks Fifth Avenue prestigious 5th Avenue Club and has been a model and spokesperson for many luxury brands. She loves to create "head to toe" exclusive imaging and styling for her clients worldwide.

Mary's humanitarian efforts and work within the not for profit world has changed the lives of thousands and create paradigm shifts in the areas of volunteerism and fundraising. She has served as President of several charities and served on many Boards of Directors. She has chaired over 100 events and produced and been creative director for equally as many in her 25 years in South Florida. She has received many awards through the years for her dedication and commitment to many charitable institutions, including "Woman of The Year", "Volunteer of the Year", 'Presidents Award", "Women of Style and Substance", "Outstanding Women of Broward County" to name a few. She also had the great privilege to Chair and Event for UNICEF and hosted Audrey Hepburn, her childhood role model. This was a dream come true!

Mary is Love In Action. No matter what medium she chooses to explore... it is unmistakably poetry and compassion. Relationships are her life and breadth. She understands and communicates the essence of relationships of all kinds and with all matter. Her gift is to explore the beauty, passion and nuances of our life experiences and share their emotional, spiritual, intellectual and physical facets in many modalities with all who seek to explore and manifest their best and most joyful lives.

Mary travel extensively, residing in Palm Beach Florida and Newport Beach California where she enjoys her children and grandchildren.

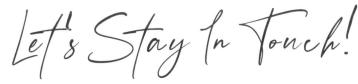

*For so much more fashion, fun, tips tricks and special offers go to:*

**www.marygiuseffi.com**

If you would like too work with me personally, or just want yo say "Hi!", please contact

**mary@marygiuseffi.com**

Find and Follow me on Facebook, Instagram and Pinterest
**Mary Giuseffi**

*To See more from my fabulous Illustrators:*

**Robin Hiers**
Robin Hiers is an artist that portrays the fun and fashionable lifestyle of beach lovers around the world. Her art is known for its sexy but playful people done with a wink and nod to the sixties.
Www.robinhiersart.com
Contact: Robinnoelart@gmail.com for inquiries

**Tracey Peer**
Tracey Peer is an impressionistic artist and travel enthusiast who captures diversified landscapes with a life full of color for all to fancy. Her artwork is sighted worldwide for its beauty, spontaneity, and vitality.
www.traceypeerart.com
Contact: traceypeerart@gmail.com for inquiries